ENERGY IS
EVERYTHING

Mindset, Nutrition & Exercise
for the best version of you

MIKE MACDONALD

To request permission for reproduction or to inquire about private coaching or speaking engagements, contact:

Mike MacDonald
Mike@AKRConditioning.com
www.MikeMacDonald.co.uk

Disclaimer
This book is not intended to provide medical advice or to take the place of medical advice and treatment from your personal physicians. Readers are advised to consult their own doctors or other qualified health professionals regarding the treatment of medical conditions. The author shall not be held liable or responsible for any misunderstanding or misuse of the information contained in this book or for any loss, damage, or injury caused or alleged to be caused directly or indirectly by any treatment, action, or application of any food or food source discussed in this book. This information is not intended to diagnose, treat, cure, or prevent any disease.

"I first met Mike MacDonald at one of my mentorships a few years back. What struck me about him was his positive energy, faith, attitude, and true desire to help people. In his new book, Energy Is Everything: Mindset, Nutrition & Exercise for the best version of you, Mike does an extraordinary job educating, motivating, and inspiring you to improve your overall health & fitness. This book is a gem that is going to truly help you live your best life. It will undoubtedly improve your health & fitness and 'Get your mind right'."

Todd Durkin, MA, CSCS
Owner, Fitness Quest 10 (San Diego, CA)
Author, The IMPACT! Body Plan
Lead Training Advisor, Under Armour

"This book makes accessible much of the academic literature on key areas of importance for active people. Written in an easy-going manner, and enriched with thought-provoking quotations from a wide literature, Mike MacDonald has brought us much more than the three themes of mind, nutrition and movement. Rather he has braided them into a strong cord which powers a lifestyle approach, which exceeds the sum of its parts. Accepting his thesis for enhancing performance, the reader can expect a range of long term dividends across a wider health domain, beyond the vanity of appearance and the preoccupation with body weight."

Dr Arthur Stewart
Institute of Health and Welfare Research
Robert Gordon University

"Mike's book is a great motivational read, based on personal experience and applied knowledge. A good tool to reinforce good nutrition and training practice."

Dr Alexandra Johnstone
Nutrition Scientist
The Rowett Institute of Nutrition and Health

Mike hits the nail on the head with "Energy Is Everything" - consistently I see the common denominator of those people that succeed in dropping weight, completing marathons or generally achieving their goals is the energy they bring to the table. To have that energy we must both be mindful in our approach to health and wellbeing but also cut ourselves some slack from time to time - being miserable because you ate a chocolate bar last night is not going to help anyone! Life is for living and energy really is everything - this book provides some great tips and advice on exercise, nutrition and wellbeing from a holistic point of view. This easy to read book is a must for anyone looking to be healthy and happy.

Louise Kochalski
Owner and Director of Training
The Health and Human Performance Centre

ABOUT THE AUTHOR

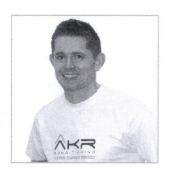

Mike MacDonald BSc, PgCert
PgCert Sports Nutrition
BSc (Hons) Sports & Exercise Science
Precision Nutrition Coach
Certified Personal Trainer
IKFF Certified Kettlebell Teacher
ISAK Level 2 Anthropometrist

Mike MacDonald is a certified personal trainer, nutrition coach, health & lifestyle blogger, and public speaker based in Aberdeen, Scotland.

A passion for football (soccer!) and a desire to enhance his own performance, inspired Mike to pursue a degree in Sports & Exercise Science. His dream of making a living from playing football didn't entirely come to fruition: Mike spent his sports career at semi-pro level, playing for 8 successful years with the Scottish Highland League team, Buckie Thistle, before a foot injury led to his retirement.

It's been said that "sometimes failing to get your goal helps you fulfill your destiny", and football (and a desire to work within football) started Mike down a path which ultimately led to him finding his passions in health & wellness and personal development. His own struggle with nutrition problems (digestive issues and binge eating) encouraged Mike to read extensively, learning everything he could about health and nutrition, behaviour change and personal development. He attained his 'Master Trainer' diploma in personal training from the European Institute of Fitness in Spain before completing the Post-Graduate Certificate in Sports Nutrition which led him to landing a dream job as Freelance Nutrition Consultant to the first team at Glasgow Rangers FC for the successful league and cup winning 2010-11 season.

ABOUT THE AUTHOR

Meanwhile, Mike continued to work as a PT at one of Scotland's premier sports facilities until in September 2011, when, after booking a one-way flight to Argentina, he resigned from his job to embark on an incredible 7-month backpacking journey throughout Latin America. Adventure apart, there was a bigger vision: the trip concluded in California where Mike was mentored by fitness industry leader, Todd Durkin, before returning home to grow his own business: AKRConditioning.

Mike feels it is important to ask for help and to seek out experts to provide it: he has also studied under internationally recognised kettlebell guru, Steve Cotter, as well as completing Dr. John Berardi's Precision Nutrition Coaching certification. He continues to be a fervent reader and blogs regularly at www.MikeMacDonald.co.uk.

ACKNOWLEDGEMENTS

I have learned so much from so many people. I am grateful to be able to draw upon the knowledge and experience of so many experts and authors who have gone before me – many of whom are referred to in this book.

On a personal level, I am especially grateful to my parents Bill and Mhairi who've both been incredibly supportive in their own ways as I took my first steps getting AKRConditioning off the ground.

I am grateful to my clients who have truly been my greatest teachers – books and theory can only take one so far. I appreciate the trust each of you placed in me as your coach, and the lessons that came with working with your individual personalities, experiences and challenges.

I owe thanks to my group of lifelong friends who've been positive about the AKRConditioning project and never failed to ask how things are going – you know who you are. Special mention to Gav for logo design, Bruce for support with those early AKR seminars, Scott for our inspiring lunchtime chats, and Lynsey for her unwavering belief in me. I'd also like to recognize the fantastic work and service of my designer Carrie@ GracelineStudios.com.

Finally, a shout out to Todd Durkin, Sean Croxton and Steve Cotter who have – without even knowing it – been role models and teachers of mine for many years. I am grateful that I was finally able to express my gratitude to each of you in person and continue to be inspired by your work. If I inspire just a fraction of the number of people you have, I'll be doing ok.

CONTENTS

FOREWORD

I first met Mike several years ago when he was working as a personal trainer at our local gym. Through hard work, vision and a passion for helping others he set up his own successful company AKRConditioning. In this book, he shares his skills and experiences, his work with clients and his understanding and interpretation of research as it applies to fitness and nutrition.

The role of the nutrition coach is to motivate clients and to provide them with relevant information on how to improve physique and performance in a healthy, sustainable and enjoyable fashion. Mike is inspirational and realistic, illustrating his approach with tales of success and lessons learned when things didn't go to plan. His book provides an excellent framework of simple strategies that can be applied to your lifestyle to improve your health, your mind-set and your body.

In the time that I have known Mike I have learned a lot from him. Now his readers have the opportunity to do the same.

Scott Baptie
Physique and sports nutrition specialist,
Director of Food For Fitness

INTRODUCTION

"Few things are sadder than encountering a person who knows exactly what he should do, yet cannot muster enough energy to do it. "He who desires but acts not," wrote Blake with his accustomed vigor, "Breeds pestilence."

(Mihaly Csikszentmihalyi, psychology professor & author,
Flow: The classic work on how to achieve happiness)

I thought I was a health freak. I'm not. I'm an energy freak. Maybe they're the same thing. Maybe not. I don't know.

All I know is that energy is everything. When we have the stuff, life is good. Without it, we suffer.

By energy, I'm not talking about fleeting highs like when your sports team wins a trophy. I'm not talking about the buzz of an extra coffee or the delight at having a long weekend off work. I'm also not talking about that person who's always 'on'. That 'bouncing off the walls', over the top, "everything's brilliant" character.

I'm talking about an overall sense of wellbeing. I'm talking about the physical energy to move gracefully through life. I'm talking about the courage to pursue what's important to us, and the spirit to get back up when life inevitably knocks us down. I'm talking about being able to thrive in life. To live it fully. To be happy. To shine. I'm talking about the ability to show up as the best version of ourselves – to be able to look, feel and perform better than we ever dreamed of.

The way I see it, our physical, mental, and emotional energy dictate the quality of our life. Although we're taught to pursue 'success' in its various forms – career, finances, relationships, physical appearance, whatever – none of these things are worth anything if they leave us without energy. You could have all the time or all the money in the world, but if your energy is in the gutter, life isn't much fun. You know what I'm talking about. There have been times you've been tired, unwell or just burnt out. There have been times you've felt depressed - weighed down by a sense of apathy. Lets be honest, if you have no energy, you have nothing. On the other hand, if you have nothing *but* great energy, you won't have nothing for long.

Energy is contagious. It attracts people and it attracts opportunities. Energy is fun. When our vibes are up, life is good. Energy ripples into every aspect of our lives: we tend to be more elegant in our relationships with others, more productive and positive at work, and still have plenty of juice in the tank to make the most of our leisure time, when we have energy. This in turn feels good, energising us some more and creating a positive cycle that allows us to continuously increase the quality of our lives. When life trips us up with one of its trusty hurdles, it's usually our energy that dictates whether or not we can dust ourselves down and keep moving forward; or whether we slide into a quiet life of desperation.

That same ripple effect exists when our energy slumps: we're not as patient, upbeat and pleasant to be around, and so our relationships suffer. We find ourselves being lazy and don't show up well at work. Our leisure time is more likely to consist of crashing in front of the TV than engaging in something that will enhance our quality of life. Since we feel low, we reach for pick-me-ups like food or alcohol which we *think* will help but which actually end up making us feel worse in the long run. We become stuck in a rut, gradually losing energy and experiencing a decreasing quality of life over time. To many, this is acceptable and we usually call it 'ageing'. To me, it's not acceptable. I want to feel good when I get up in the morning. I want to feel great. Energy is everything.

I didn't think it was always like this but, looking back, maybe it kinda was. Football was my life, and I wanted to improve my performance. To become better. I guess you could say that even then it was really about having more energy. I studied sports and exercise science. I was a semi-pro trying to eat and prepare as a pro would. Really, I was an amateur. Despite enjoying a successful football career, I never made the grade. Worse, I never fulfilled my potential. I always felt I was capable of more. If only I knew what I know now.

I graduated and got a job in corporate health and fitness. I started working with real people. Trying to help. At the same time, I was still trying to be the best footballer I could. I'd had a couple of bad injuries. My legs always felt tight. My digestion wasn't great. I frequently felt bloated and was lethargic at times. So I dived deeper into health and nutrition (some of my friends might say I dived too deep!). I devoured books on the topic and became a personal trainer. Working with real people – including myself –

highlighted the importance of mindset. Of motivation and behaviour change. Of habits. So I studied that too.

While I'm no guru, I have learned a lot. From experts who've travelled this way before me. From my own challenges. From my clients. And although there is a natural ebb and flow to things in life, in general my energy is strong. I feel good when I wake up. This matters to me because just as my football career came to an end, I know one day my life will too. This time I don't want to get to the end feeling that I was capable of more. I want to be the best version of myself. I want the same for you. Life is short. Regardless of your goal, regardless of whether or not you are a big dreamer, you might as well squeeze the juice out of life. You might as well be happy. You might as well look, feel and perform at your best. After all, potential unexpressed turns to pain.

Perhaps you feel you've tried all this 'health stuff' before. I thought I had too. I was wrong, and having great energy isn't just about eating less and exercising more. The chances are you already know some of the things you 'should' be doing. I'm not just going to tell you to eat your greens and get some exercise. You already know that stuff. Becoming the best version of you starts with an area almost entirely neglected by fitness pros and diet gurus – the mind. So Part One of this book addresses mindset. You'll learn how to feel better *now* by thinking in ways that help rather than hinder you. You'll see why the typical health kick is usually short-lived and learn a more effective route to lasting change. We'll tackle the motivation issue – why the old model of motivation doesn't work and what you can do to do fire yourself up.

Part Two centres on nutrition. You already know it's important. We'll look at why it's so confusing and why it so often ends in disaster. Rather than just tell you *what* to do, I'll actually share the practical 'hows' of helpful eating, and discuss the challenges so many of us face around eating behaviour. There's more to it than food though. We'll also be looking at the other oft-neglected means of nourishing ourselves that have a huge impact on our quality of life.

Part Three is about exercise. It's another area where the mainstream model is a little flawed. Most of us are doing it wrong ...or not at all. I hope to offer you a new perspective of exercise. Of course I'll also discuss how to exercise for fat loss. We complete the loop by returning to the mind and the importance of exercising our brain.

It is my hope that you find this book practical, insightful and encouraging. It contains the hours of reading and studying I've done. It contains the lessons from my own journey and the hours in the field with real clients. It contains the mindset, nutrition and exercise strategies you need to be the best version of you.

Energy is everything.

Mike

PART ONE >

Mindset

Usually when people come to me for help improving the way they look, feel and perform in life, they want to dive straight into nutrition and exercise: what to eat, what not to eat, what the best training programme is. Of course that stuff is important, but without first addressing our *mindset* – the way we think and what we believe – it's likely that this latest health kick (or any other self-improvement project), will turn out to be just as short-lived as it's predecessors did: you're not the only one who has tried before.

Addressing mindset makes all the difference. Get your mind right, and the rest will follow. One of the most crucial insights regarding mindset is *choice*.

CHOICE

"Everything can be taken from a man but one thing: to choose one's attitudes in any given set of circumstances, to choose one's own way"

(Viktor Frankl, neurologist, psychiatrist & Holocaust survivor)

Viktor Frankl survived a Nazi concentration camp. *By choice.* It wasn't that he simply chose to survive when others chose to die. He survived by finding meaning in the unspeakable suffering he was made to endure. He survived by *choosing his thoughts*.

Everything starts with thoughts. Our thoughts dictate our feelings, and our feelings drive our actions. The actions we take (or don't take) determine our outcomes – in this case: how we look, feel and perform in life. So, if we are to make a change in our lives, we have to begin with our thoughts. Although we all have the power to choose our thoughts, most of us live on autopilot with our lives at the whim of external circumstances: stuff happens, it makes us feel something (which we label 'good' or 'bad') and we react. Thoughts control emotions, emotions dictate energy, and energy drives actions. When I broke my foot, I perceived it as bad and I felt depressed. I lacked the energy to be patient and I snapped at people I care about. Autopilot. I reacted. So rather than cruising along on autopilot and letting external circumstances dictate our energy, the first step is to understand this:

Nothing has any meaning of its own.
Meaning is something we attach to things by thinking about them.

"Things cannot touch the mind: they are external and inert;
anxieties can only come from your external judgment."
(Marcus Aurelius, Roman emperor & philosopher)

I find it curious that many people describe weather as "miserable" (it happens a lot here in Scotland!) Weather isn't miserable; weather is weather. As novelist Paul Theroux writes, *"only a fool blames his bad vacation on the rain."* We might feel miserable because it's raining outside but that's down to our *perception* of the weather. For some, the rain might be a blessing. Back when I played football, I much preferred playing the game on drizzly Saturday afternoon than on hot and dry one. I also know some people who love nothing better than being wrapped up warm, watching a movie while the rain thunders down outside. Some people love the rain! By the same token, nothing is inherently sad, nothing is inherently frustrating, and nothing is inherently boring. Nothing is, by its nature, exciting or fun. These are all merely labels we use to describe things based upon our perception of them. Don't believe me? How come some people find public speaking to be a thrill, while for others it's the scariest thing imaginable? Some see golf as an addictive, absorbing, fun and interesting sport, whereas others will tell you it's a frustrating, boring, pointless game. What's the truth? Who is correct? Neither. Golf is golf.

Am I saying that we should put the blinkers on and perceive everything as hunky-dory all the time? No, of course not. We all face challenging times, we all feel sadness and get depressed from time to time. It's normal. We live in a world of complimentary opposites: light and dark, up and down, hot and cold. Without one side, the other cannot exist – we need some sadness to know what happiness is. Therefore, in this world of duality, a negative cannot exist without a positive and more often than not, our greatest gifts and lessons come from our most challenging experiences. Without the foot injury I mentioned earlier – a misdiagnosed mess that eventually led to my premature retirement from football – I'd probably still be playing in the semi-pro 'bubble', closed off from the host of new experiences and opportunities I've had since.

> *"Opportunities to find deeper powers within ourselves*
> *come when life seems most challenging."*
> *(Joseph Campbell, mythologist, writer & lecturer)*

Even in situations like death, positives can be found – if we're courageous enough to look. Death brings people together, and in connecting people to their own sense of mortality, a death can spark a sense of urgency: it helps us to realise what's truly important in life – death is what makes life precious! Challenging circumstances are what help us to grow and develop our character. If we want to be strong or brave or compassionate, we have to experience situations that require strength or bravery or compassion. Coming out stronger is the prize. On the other hand, when life is too easy, by default it becomes hard. Everybody knows of a child who experiences too much support and not enough challenge: they grow up unable to do anything for themselves. No, the tough times, the challenges, are absolutely necessary in life and when we realise that they always carry something positive – even if that positive takes years to reveal itself – we can learn to perceive them in a more helpful manner. We can learn optimism.

> *"Optimism is realizing that the more painful the event, the more profound the lesson.*
> *Once you bring this knowledge into your heart, you can never again look at any event as*
> *all bad. Optimism gives you power over fear of the future and regret for the past."*
> *(Baker & Stauth, authors, What Happy People Know)*

Given that fear and regret are the primary forces that hold us back from our best selves, this understanding of optimism goes a long way in helping us to perceive the events of our lives in more helpful ways.

SILENCING 'THE CHIMP'

The next step is to switch off our autopilot and take control of our perceptions. To do this, to choose our thoughts, we must first become aware of them. We must be aware of 'The Chimp' in our head – the one that's usually wreaking havoc and telling us rubbish that doesn't serve us. The self-defeating statements, the "what-if's", the irrational fears, and the stories we tell ourselves all come from The Chimp: most of us are so used to him or her swinging around in there that we don't recognise the negativity that's polluting our mind and crushing our energy. Our brain is designed for survival and while fearful, negative thoughts might keep us safe, they often prevent us from thriving. Don't believe every thought you have!

"I've had thousands of problems in my life, most of which never happened."

(Mark Twain, author)

When we become aware of our thoughts, we can start to take control of that inner Chimp. Rather than reacting like a chimp, we can respond: we can choose a thought which serves us, one that will protect our energy. We can make a mountain out of a molehill, or a molehill out of a mountain. One of the best ways to do this is to ask ourselves quality questions. Consider the difference between our usual 'chimp chatter' and the quality questions in the table on the next page.

CHIMP CHATTER	QUALITY QUESTIONS
I can't believe this happened!	What's good about this?
If only I hadn't...	How does this serve me?
Why do I always...?	What can I learn from this?
I can't believe they did that to me!	What else could this mean?
Oh my god oh my god oh my god!	What's important here?
I need ice-cream/chocolate/alcohol!	What can I do to make me feel better?
I'm such a loser/I'm disgusting/what a fatty/etc.	What can I do about this? (focus on what you want vs what you don't want)
I can't	How can I?
Worst. Day. Ever.	What can I appreciate right now?
(any time we catch ourselves 'sweating the small stuff')	Will I care about this tomorrow/next week/3 months from now?

Ultimately, our energy, our life, is determined not by what happens, but how we think about what happens. It's possible to perceive the same event or the same circumstances in very different ways just by changing the questions we ask and the stories we tell ourselves. In *What Happy People Know*, Baker & Stauth share the three main mistakes we make when it comes to perception:

1. **Permanence.** We think that the problem will last forever. It seldom does. In fact, often the things that we let upset us will be completely forgotten the next day!

2. **Personalisation.** We believe every problem is our own fault. It's always about us. This is a sign of playing the victim. In reality, no one is out to get us. If someone else is rude or unkind, more often than not it's about him or her rather than us. Maybe that person is having a bad day!

3. **Pervasiveness.** We think that one problem extends to every other situation in life. Rarely is this the case.

With this awareness, we can choose to take responsibility for our thoughts and choose thoughts that will help; or we can play the victim and choose thoughts that hinder. If Viktor Frankl could demonstrate that very power, in the midst of experiencing some of the worst horrors imaginable in a Nazi concentration camp, then each of us is capable of doing the same in our own lives.

HABITS

As we know, *choosing* to do something, however, isn't enough. Actually taking the action to get it done, is something different altogether. The majority of us already know some of the behaviours that are limiting our energy and our results, and we know at least *some* things we could do to improve things. We could decide to silence The Chimp, or decide to eat well or start exercising, but unless these things become habitual, we'll keep taking one step forward and two back. This is because rather than one-off actions, epiphanies or events, it's our habits which shape our lives. Those seemingly inconsequential actions that we do consistently, soon add up. No one gets out of shape overnight. Many of us though, realise that several years have passed and that habitual muffin with the coffee, that regular nibbling in the evenings, or that customary beer or two to unwind after work have 'suddenly' made a huge difference to the way we look, feel and perform. It's funny that: habits seem to work with a bit of stealth – they seem so inconsequential in the moment that we don't notice their impact until years pass by and we're either in a rut or we're living our dreams. This is because, in the moment, we're often not even aware of them:

"When a habit emerges, the brain stops fully participating in decision making. It stops working so hard, or diverts focus to other tasks. So, unless you deliberately fight a habit – unless you find new routines – the pattern will unfold automatically."
(Charles Duhigg, author, The Power of Habit)

It's *automatic*: the way we think, speak and act all become unconscious habits. The good news is that habits can be positive as well as negative. Just as we all learned to form the habit of cleaning our teeth, people with great energy tend to have made a habit of silencing The Chimp. It becomes normal for them to ask quality questions, to seek, and to find, the opportunities and the blessings that come hidden in every challenge. Likewise, people who are in great shape are usually those who've made a habit of exercising and eating well – it becomes a ritual and, like cleaning your teeth: It. Just.

Gets. Done. Magnified by time, these tiny habits and others (like saving a little money each month, reading a little, planning the day ahead, or simply smiling some more!) stack up to completely transform our energy and our life.

What if you made a habit of being your own cheerleader rather than constantly self-criticising? What if you automatically started your workouts, right on cue – be it morning, lunchtime or evenings? What if, instead of the beers, it became routine for you to unwind each evening by practising a musical instrument or learning something new for 15 minutes? What if you cultivated the habit of planning your day: getting up early, recommitting to what matters, deciding on the few most important things to be done, and doing them? What would that do for your life?

"There's nothing you can't do if you get the habits right."
(Charles Duhigg, author, The Power of Habit)

Once we recognise that habits are vital, we can learn to focus on *behaviours* rather than *outcomes*. Behaviours – eating vegetables every day – we can control; outcomes – the number on the scales – we can't.

The next step then, is to begin cultivating behaviours that will help us. Habits can be tricky things to form and to break and unfortunately, this is where many of us get it wrong. Here's what we usually do: for some reason or another, we find ourselves motivated to change. Maybe we've got a holiday coming up or a wedding, or maybe it's January – the official health kick time of year. Regardless, we're fed up of our current state and are ready to act. We dive into healthy eating and exercise. Fantastic! But... as we know all too well, after only a few weeks of action we find ourselves back at square one. Only 12% of us who make New Years resolutions actually achieve our goal.[1] I'm not convinced that this is because we're all lazy, stupid or weak-willed. This is about habits.

Consider the typical person starting a health kick. Changing what they eat involves changing their shopping habits, their cooking habits, the actual foods they eat, and the tastes and textures they're accustomed to. This person might choose to make a habit of keeping a food journal or at least eating more mindfully and at consistent times. They also have to break the habit of snacking on lower quality foods, which can be a huge challenge in itself. At the same time, they've probably decided to start exercising

...another new habit. A habit which might also require the habit of actually getting themselves to the gym – if it's before work, then they might need to form the habit of getting up earlier; if it's after work, habitual mealtimes may change. Of course they'll need to get into the habit of taking their gym kit with them to work, and get used to the change in physical sensations that come with exercise. All of this is likely to necessitate a change in schedule and most likely the habit of planning in advance. So, in order to be able to get up earlier, or prepare their food or gym kit for the day ahead, they'll need to sacrifice some leisure time activities – like that late-night TV habit. Moreover, these changes could also mean a change for other people in the household. Will that be greeted with resistance or support? This brings us to the habits of the mental game. Our person will need to practice being disciplined when they don't feel like it rather than the habit of justifying old behaviours with the "I'll start Monday" mantra. They might also need to practice the habit of acting in the face of fear or resistance. Leaving a comfort zone – be it physically, through exercise – or socially, through joining a new club, is a requirement for growth, and you can bet there'll be peer pressure and plenty of 'crabs in the barrel* trying to pull them back to old ways.

Ok, maybe I'm sensationalising a little. Maybe. But the point is that the 'simple changes' we're so often advised to make, might actually require a boatload of behaviour change, and while some people are able to make huge shifts with seemingly relative ease (more on that later), for most of us, trying to change more than one habit at a time is the very reason we fail. So rather than surfing a wave of motivation until the next inevitable wipeout, we'd be wise to adopt a more patient approach and narrow our focus to just one thing at a time. According to Leo Babauta, writer of the top ten blog, *Zen Habits*, doing so increases our rate of success from 0% (when we try to change multiple habits at once) to up to 80% - provided we follow some rules:

* We focus on one new habit at a time (this lets us narrow our focus).
* The habit change should be easier than we think we can handle – thus ensuring and reinforcing success (which we can build on later).
* The habit change should be measureable (did I do it today - yes or no?).
* The habit change should – as far as possible – be done at a consistent time each day. This helps to develop a trigger for the desired behaviour.
* We record daily. Checking-in on a daily basis is a great way to keep the habit in mind, and keep ourselves accountable.
* We stay positive. Expect occasional setbacks, learn from them, adopt a 'clean slate' policy and move on.

---

* From Wikipedia: *"The metaphor refers to a pot of crabs. Individually, the crabs could easily escape from the pot, but instead, they grab at each other in a useless "king of the hill" competition which prevents any from escaping and ensures their collective demise. The analogy in human behavior is that members of a group will attempt to "pull down" (negate or diminish the importance of) any member who achieves success beyond the others, out of envy, conspiracy or competitive feelings."* http://en.wikipedia.org/wiki/Crab_mentality

If we return to our typical person above, in practice this might mean putting the exercise regime and healthy diet on hold for the meantime, and focussing solely on developing the habit of eating mindfully (sitting down, distraction-free, and slowly chewing and enjoying their meal). To make this habit measureable, a simple target of ensuring that mealtimes last 15 minutes could be set. To record their new habit, our person could cross off a day on their calendar or even record it with their smartphone (yes, there are apps for that!). If 15 minutes seemed a stretch, they could shoot for 10 minutes, or apply the habit only for their evening meal. Once this 'new normal' has been established (on average 66 days - but anything from 18 to 254 days[2]) our person could start thinking about adding a habit based around the type of foods they eat (although, just by eating slowly, they'll probably find that they've spontaneously started making better food choices already – without even trying!).

I get that this approach may seem very pedantic – especially at times like in January when we're champing at the bit to get going – but if we can rein ourselves in, we'll find that slow change is longer lasting. We stay the course. Rather than those repeated stop-start cycles in which we might change a little but don't or can't sustain it, the slow approach allows us to gather momentum and continually build on a series of previous mini-wins. What sort of difference could a few helpful habits consistently built up over several years make in your life? And we all agree that time flies anyway so what's the rush? The last five years of my life have passed in the blink of an eye. I'm finding that really *there is no short-term*. We have the present moment in which we can act, and we have the long-term: when all those little present-moment actions have compounded on each other to produce a positive or negative result.

"Your only path to success is through a continuum of mundane, unsexy, unexciting, and sometimes difficult daily disciplines compounded over time."
(Darren Hardy, author & publisher of SUCCESS Magazine)

On the other hand, when we do rush, we get seduced by 'solutions'. There is always something: new diets, supplements and 'superfoods'; new exercise products and programmes, or new technology that we believe holds the answer – that "this time" it'll be different – but unless that solution addresses the habit (which pretty much none of them do) we'll continue flip-flopping from one thing to the next. This is why so many people, myself included, have at least one piece of exercise equipment currently gathering dust in their home. The new 'thing' isn't the answer – committing to doing the fundamentals, consistently, over time is. Habits are.

MOTIVATION

"In some cases, success is less about hard work, resources, and skill, and more about motivation. Sometimes you have to find the right incentives that push you and drive you before you can reach your dreams."

(Eric Thomas, speaker, educator & author)

Of course the slow approach still requires effort – which we can choose to perceive as a good thing! After all, there's little reward to be had without having overcome some sort of challenge. Trouncing my 7-year-old nephew in a game of pool, for instance, yields little satisfaction (it didn't please him much either!) Without at least *some* effort, there is no sense of accomplishment, no feeling of fulfilment. The question is: how do we stay motivated to keep putting in consistent effort over a sustained period of time? How do we keep going in the face of adversity, when we don't see results and it no longer seems like fun?

The conventional approach to motivation is the old carrot and stick method of reward and punishment. This approach is rife in health and fitness: "if I exercise today I can eat that piece of chocolate". Or, "if I eat too much, I'll have to hammer the treadmill tomorrow". Not only is trading food for exercise somewhat flawed logic, as Daniel Pink explains in his book *Drive: The surprising truth about what motivates us*, rather than encourage us, these kind of 'if-then' rewards actually tend to "extinguish" motivation and promote short-term thinking. Even when we adopt the longer-term, habit-based model of building momentum, the carrot and stick approach doesn't seem to cut it. We face strong temptations on a daily basis and punishments, "my doctor says I'm at high-risk for heart-disease" (i.e. I might die!), and rewards, "so I can look good on holiday", aren't enough to keep us on track. But you already know that from your own experiences. If they were, I'd become a travel agent: anytime anyone wanted to get themselves in shape, I'd just tell them to book a beach holiday!

Don't get me wrong, external incentives can play a role – having a coach or mentor to report to and hold us accountable can have a dramatic effect on our adherence when it comes to habit-building, and I'm a big proponent of finding some kind of social support. However, even with those things in place, we'll have limited success without considering the inner game.

AUTONOMY

"The science shows that the secret to high performance isn't our biological drive or our reward-and-punishment drive, but our third drive – our deep-seated desire to direct our own lives, to extend and expand our abilities, and to live a life of purpose".

(Daniel Pink, author, Drive: The surprising truth about what motivates us)

Rather than build a new habit to please our doctor, or try to improve the way we look because we feel we *have* to in order to satisfy our spouse or societal ideals, Pink shows that motivation is best when we feel a sense of *autonomy*. That is, having a level of freedom over the activity and taking ownership of it: being able to choose what we do, when we do it, with whom, and how. The project is our own.

Imagine a group of schoolchildren are painting pictures of animals. One class is given a painting-by-numbers task with no choice over what animal is to be painted or how – just paint the elephant grey. The other class is invited to paint any animal they wish, with any colours and any style of their choosing. Which class do you think will be most motivated? Where will we see the most inspiration, the hardest work – irrespective of external grades or rewards? At some point in your life you've been given a project at school or work where the rules are hard and fast: "this is *what* needs to be done, and this is *how* it needs to be done." It's like painting by numbers and – for most people – it's not a particularly inspiring proposition. In fact, it's probably a chore – even if there is a big reward waiting at the end of it. Incredibly, even when the reward is *life* itself, people tend not to be particularly motivated when they're 'told' what to do. The World Health Organisation estimates that only about 50% of patients with chronic diseases actually follow treatment recommendations[3]. Compare that with a project of your own choosing, a project which, within a certain framework, you have some creative freedom. These are the kind of projects that we find ourselves immersed in, that we're motivated to work on – even after work. This is why we see computer programmers who are demotivated at work (despite their rewarding salary) come home and spend hours designing a website or an app – for free!

Having some sense of ownership over the task lets us do things from choice rather than obligation. It becomes "I *want* to" or "I *get* to", instead of "I *should*" or "I *ought* to". With this mindset, it becomes much easier to follow through. This mindset also lets us tap into the concept of *mastery*: a devotion to our craft.

MASTERY

"The quality of a person's life is in direct proportion to their commitment to excellence, regardless of their chosen field of endeavour."
(Vince Lombardi, American football coach)

Mastery is a commitment to excellence in which the reward is the activity itself. We forget about 'motivation' as such, and just get immersed in our task. It becomes absorbing and addictive as we continually fine-tune things, improving as we go. It's mastery that's at work when we see people become enthralled by projects – it could be a sport, a musical instrument or even a project for work. I see it all the time when people get the 'gym bug' – they start to improve the way their body looks and functions, and get captivated by that improvement. Motivation isn't an issue – sometimes time even goes out the window. When I was younger I loved to practice 'keepie uppie' – juggling the football and working on my technique. I could spend hours at it – hours that would pass in minutes. I was 'in the zone', a state of *flow* described by Mihaly Csikszentmihalyi in his book *Flow: The classic work on how to achieve happiness*, as the key to happiness. We do it for the sake of doing it.

In a health and fitness context, I've seen clients inspired by a journey of mastering cookery. I've seen friends become absorbed in improving their ability at new sports like climbing or surfing, and I know bodybuilders who just love to manipulate and master the way their body looks. Indeed, any project undertaken in this way – be it at work or play – is likely to energise us. But what if enhancing your energy really does depend on implementing some health and fitness changes, and mastery in that area of your life just doesn't fire you up? Instead of catching the gym bug, the gym just bugs you.
Well... what you need is a 'why'. We all do.

OUR 'WHY'

*"The successful person has the habit of doing the things failures don't like to do.
They don't like doing them either necessarily.
But their disliking is subordinated to the strength of their purpose."*

(Albert E.N. Gray, author)

Reasons precede results. Our 'why' is our missing link to motivation. Steven Covey, who wrote the famous, *The 7 Habits of Highly Effective People*, tells us that *"happiness can be defined, in part at least, as the fruit of the desire and ability to sacrifice what we want now for what we want eventually"*. Great. But given the temptations we all face on a daily basis, unless we've got an inspiring *why*, a compelling reason to do so, we'll find it difficult to repeatedly make that sacrifice. You know very well that we tend to choose what feels good in the moment.

If you're like me, you might notice that sometimes you are fired up, enthusiastic, focussed, inspired, and nothing's going to get in the way of your goals - it's easy to make the smart choices. We are 'in state': the best possible frame of mind. Other times though, we're not feeling it as much: the path of least resistance is the one that's most appealing. Even though we know we'll feel worse in the long run, we just feel like vegging out. We know what choice would better serve our goals, but we can't get ourselves to do it. We're in a state! Knowing isn't enough. Being rational only helps to a point. Motivation is fuelled by emotion. So obviously we want to get ourselves 'in state' as often as possible. How do we do that? Our why. Or even a list of whys. Whatever it is, it must *mean* something to us – it must generate some emotion or feeling, it's got to fire us up!

With a deep sense of purpose on our side, we're able to endure a lot more struggle and sometimes even make huge shifts in an instant. I always remember my guidance teacher at school telling us that for years he tried and failed to give up smoking. Then he had a throat cancer scare and never touched a cigarette again. Reasons precede results.

Now we're not all likely to experience a life-changing epiphany like that, but with a bit of introspection, we can find a strong emotional reason to drive us toward our goals. I know what you're thinking: you already have a why. People are sick and tired of being sick and tired and I see folks in the gym who're *desperate* to lose weight. I've had clients who "need" to get in shape for their holiday and there're plenty of guys out there who believe that if they can just get six-pack abs, all of life's woes will evaporate in an instant. These are nice incentives – to look good, to feel good, to be more confident – but they're easily forgotten in the tough moments, on our down days. It's too easy to rationalise skipping that workout today (we'll make up for it, right?), and as good as looking great on holiday will feel, that's off in the future, and eating that Danish pastry looks pretty good RIGHT NOW!

Our why needs to be bigger than that. Ideally it involves something bigger than ourselves: making a difference, a contribution – a higher purpose. Often it's tied to what's truly most important in our life.

Take, for example, a young mother who is inconsistent with her health goals. Like many, she struggles to stay motivated, repeating that familiar stop-start cycle over and over again. Every time she starts over, it's with the promise that "this time it's different", and with every failure comes even more heartache and loss of self-esteem. Sooner or later she gives up – at some level she labels herself 'broken': lacking willpower and self-discipline. When we look at her life, however, we find that when it comes to her kids, it's a different story altogether. If the kids are sick, she's there. If the kids need a lift home, done. She makes all manner of sacrifices to be able to take the kids on exciting holidays, to buy them nice clothes and to make their dreams come true at Christmas. She'll get up early to pack their lunches and stay up late having helped them with their homework. Clearly she doesn't lack willpower or self-discipline at all. She's not broken; with the right why (the wellbeing of her kids) she can do *anything*, she's superwoman! In fact, in 2006, a mother was even reported to have fought off a polar bear to protect her 7-year-old son![4] Albeit anecdotal, stories of people who've demonstrated 'impossible' feats – like Lauren Kornacki, who apparently lifted a car to save her dad who was trapped underneath – show the power of purpose. "My dad means everything to me," Lauren said[5].

What does your goal mean to you? How badly do you want it?

For big goals, we need 'gazelle intensity', a concept introduced by financial author Dave Ramsay. We all know that the cheetah is the fastest animal on earth but did you know that on average it only catches the gazelle once in every nineteen attempts?[†] Not only can the gazelle outmanoeuvre the cheetah, but he also has more focus: the cheetah is running for a meal; the gazelle is running for his life!

† As reported by Dave Ramsey in 'The Total Money Makeover Workbook'

Improving your health and your energy might not mean the life or death of you or a loved one, but if we can find a way to link our goal to what's most important in our life we might just find some gazelle intensity of our own. I'd ask our young mother to write down 50 reasons why her being healthier will benefit her kids. Suddenly it's not about herself anymore and she's fired up about eating well and exercising so that she can be a better mother. Purpose. Meaning. A why.

A guy called Eric Thomas provides us with another example. Eric grew up in the ghettos of Detroit, was a high school dropout and homeless for a time. It took him *12 years* to get his 4-year degree but at the time of writing he's on the verge of achieving his PhD and has become a prominent motivational speaker and author. You don't show Eric's kind of grit without a big why. Eric's why is to inspire underprivileged kids from tough backgrounds like his own, "to be a champion for the underdog", as he puts it. "If I can do it" Eric says, "anyone can".

Finding our why isn't necessarily easy or straightforward: it's a process that might take some time. Sometimes it means going deep! Go easy on yourself though, while some people just know or stumble upon their calling, for others it might take a lot of introspection. It's also likely to change a little throughout your life. Like Eric Thomas, people often become inspired about helping others through some difficulty they've struggled with in their own life – it's the classic example of turning a challenge into a gift. A useful exercise is to ask ourselves "how bad do you want it?" and then follow up with "why?" to every answer that we come up with – in that slightly irritating manner a small child does. This process is akin to unpeeling an onion: we remove layer after layer and go deeper and deeper until we get close to our true reason. It's amazing what can happen. What was initially about losing fat can become about our legacy or making a difference in world or in the lives of others. It's so much easier when it's not just about us. This is how ordinary and often relatively out-of-shape folks pull themselves through marathons – often they're raising money for a cause that is dear to their heart. Am I suggesting that we need to know the meaning of life before we make any improvement? No, just that <u>emotion fuels motivation</u> and the bigger the emotional driver – the bigger the why – the better.

Here are some some other questions that might help.

What do I want? How bad do I want it? Why?
What do I react to? What inspires me, saddens me, makes me angry?
When I was a child, what did I want to be when I grew up?
If money was meaningless, what would I do with my life?
Where in my life am I most disciplined?
What do I think or dream about most?
How would I like to be remembered when I die?
What fires me up?
Where do I get lost in the moment?
Why do I get out of bed in the morning?
What would get me out of bed in the morning?

If you wrote a list of whys that truly fired you up, that put you 'in state' and looked at that list –
and maybe even some inspiring pictures – on a daily basis, what might that do for your ability to stay on track?

"Discipline is remembering what you want."
(David Campbell, author)

It starts with why.

PART ONE SUMMARY

- Everything starts in the mind.
- Thoughts lead to emotions, emotions lead to actions, actions determine results.
- Nothing has any intrinsic meaning of it's own.
- We can choose our thoughts and the way we perceive life's events.
- We live in a world of duality: every challenge carries something good.
- Asking quality questions helps offer another perspective.
- Our energy is determined by our habits: the small things we do consistently over time.
- We can only control behaviours; we cannot control outcomes.
- Focussing on one easy habit change at a time produces best results.
- Take a slow, long-term approach, and focus on the fundamentals.
- Quick fixes and 'solutions' don't work because they neglect habit change.
- A sense of accomplishment requires effort.
- Consistent effort requires motivation.
- The punishment-reward theory of motivation is limited.
- Having a sense of autonomy over our projects fuels our motivation.
- A commitment to mastery is important: finding joy in the task for its own sake.
- Everybody needs a 'why': an emotional reason to drive us on.

PART TWO >

Nutrition

Getting our mind right goes a long way to improving our energy. It's the key, first step that most of us neglect. Choosing thoughts and questions that help rather than hinder us, focussing on fundamental habits and finding our motivation, really are game-changers when it comes to becoming the best version of ourselves.

But... we cannot fuel ourselves on good vibes alone. So as well as our mind, we must nourish our body.

FOOD CONFUSION

"Perhaps some foods really are better than others. But we are not mice in a laboratory. We are complex human beings, and we are also really prone to being dead wrong with our seemingly-genius-at-the-time beliefs about what is and is not good for us."

(Matt Stone, author Diet Recovery 2)

What we eat affects *everything*. What we eat has a dramatic impact on our day-to-day energy levels. What we eat influences how we *look*: our body composition of fat and muscle as well as the quality of our skin, teeth, eyes and hair. What we eat influences how we *feel*: our health in general – pain, inflammation, allergies and the development of chronic diseases, as well as our sleep, our alertness and our ability to concentrate. What we eat also influences how we *perform* physically: in day-to-day life and in our exercise pursuits – whatever the level of competition. What we eat impacts our hormones and our genetic expression – perhaps even the genes we pass on to our great grandchildren! How's that for legacy? (Check out *Deep Nutrition* by Catherine & Luke Shanahan for a detailed discussion of this.) While there are those who may be completely unattached to what they eat; for most of us, food also has a powerful emotional component: it can be highly rewarding, it affects our mood, and tends to be an important feature of our social lives: connecting, sharing, and 'breaking bread' with others. There are also issues like the environment: sustainability, food miles, food waste, farming practices, and the treatment of animals. There's the business and politics of the food industry as well as food science and genetic engineering. There's international trade and world hunger. These all affect economics, markets and wider issues in the world. Like it or not, food is kind of a big deal! No wonder many people treat it like a religion!

What to eat can be a complicated and confusing topic. Healthy eating means a lot of different things to a lot of different people. The mainstream approach (led by the food companies) promotes the idea that saturated fat is bad and it's all about a "balanced" diet and getting your "5-a-day" of fruit and vegetables (or any product that has the slightest resemblance to fruit or vegetable!) Low-fat, low calorie products are heralded as the route to weight loss. 'Special K' anyone? Or of course anything that comes in green-coloured packaging and has one of a thousand different health claims. That *must* be good for us!

Then we have the ever-growing fringe groups: some people feel great on a vegan diet. Other people change their lives by adopting a 'paleo' diet. Some people get best results eating 6-8 small meals a day; others swear by a 'warrior diet' of only one large meal per day, or for periodically skipping an entire day of eating. For some, being a 'raw foodie' is the answer. For others it's juicing. There are people out there who advocate a low-fat diet. There are people who feel best eating 70-80% of their diet from fat. Some people eat low-carb; others eat high-carb or practice 'carb cycling' or 'carb backloading'. Some people optimise things by weighing and measuring: meticulously tracking every morsel of food that crosses their lips. Others wing it. Some have 'cheat days' or 'reward' meals. Others religiously eat 'clean'. Some avoid gluten or dairy or eggs or soy or nuts or fish. Others eat whatever they wish. Aaargh! It's exasperating just writing this!

Nutrition is confusing because to some extent everything works. There are people thriving with each of the above eating styles. There are vegan powerlifters, paleo marathon runners and everything in between. Then there are those folks who could seemingly eat a bucket of nails and still do great! Back when I played football, two of the leanest, fittest players on the team had – by most people's standards – the worst diet. We'd be on the train at 7.30am ahead of a gruelling journey to play later that afternoon and my teammate would be tucking into a breakfast of sweets and crisps. Seriously. ... Oh, and he sported a six-pack and was consistently one of our best performers (don't you just love those guys!).

Amidst these contradictory experiences and the onslaught of conflicting information, we commonly fall into a couple of traps. One, we confuse *correlation* with *causation*: we assume that because someone behaves a certain way (i.e. eats a certain diet) and has a favourable outcome (i.e. looks, feels or performs well), that person's particular behaviour is *causing* the desired outcome. It goes like this, for example:

> Bodybuilders are lean and muscular.
> Bodybuilders consume protein shakes.
> Protein shakes make bodybuilders lean and muscular.

But we've jumped the gun a little here - there are of course several different things that contribute to the physique of the bodybuilder. It sounds obvious I know, but intelligent people make this sort of assumption repeatedly in "peer-reviewed" academic journals. The classic example is that people with heart disease often have high cholesterol – true. Therefore high cholesterol causes heart disease. Not true. Not true at all[6,7,8,9,10,11]. That's like saying every time it rains I see people with umbrellas; therefore people with umbrellas cause rain. Clearly this is absurd! Still, we take it further by making the second assumption that because something works for someone else, it will work for us. Bill skips breakfast every day and has great results; so to get great results, I should start skipping breakfast. This is also a mistake.

How come? Because we're all different. We have different start points: different states of health, physiology and function. We have different hormonal statuses; different body compositions or body types; different genetic tendencies and different responses to foods. We live different lifestyles in different environments. We sleep different amounts; have different psychological dispositions and different stress levels - or different abilities to manage stress. We have different goals and different hobbies and different exercise habits. We are exposed to different influences and have different belief systems regarding food behaviours and reward – some of us were trained to "clear the plate because there are children starving in Ethiopia", others that "it's polite to leave some food on the side". Some can be rational about food as 'fuel'; others grew up emotionally tied to the idea of food as a reward, or attached to fond memories like baking cookies with Grandma. Lots of wildly different things work for different people. What we need to remember is that just because eating style 'x' worked for someone else doesn't necessarily mean it will work for us.

Another problem is the tribalism around nutrition. What we eat can dramatically alter our lives and when people find an eating style that works wonders for them, they understandably want to tell the world about it. Unfortunately, what starts with some well-intentioned enthusiasm often becomes an increasingly dogmatic, cultish, and religious approach to eating. Yes, food choices have far reaching consequences but it's easy to become neurotic. Regardless of our food beliefs or eating style, food snobbery or casting judgement upon others for their food choices doesn't help anyone. It's a shame to see so many health and fitness professionals and researchers indulge in petty games of one-upmanship that do nothing but cause further food confusion – especially when, with a desire to help others, they're all meant to be on the same team!

What we need is a common starting point. What are the fundamentals?

NOURISHMENT

> *"We needn't scratch our heads wondering which fad diet we should follow and which – because experts now say so – we should reject."*
> (Catherine Shanahan, author Deep Nutrition)

Nutrition – food! – is about *nourishment*. Regardless of our goal – whether it's weight-loss, doing a mud run, being a competitive sportsperson, or merely enjoying great energy – we must start by nourishing our body. It's that simple.

I have worked with many clients who act as if undernourishment (starvation) is the key to weight loss. It's not their fault: the 'eat less, exercise more' dogma runs strong in our society, it's deeply ingrained in our social conditioning. If we can work out, endure hunger and resist the body's natural urge to eat, we're *bound* to be successful! Yet, without adequate nutrients: the vitamins, minerals, enzymes, proteins, fats, carbohydrates and water – all required at a cellular level – our body cannot possibly function at it's best. As Sean Croxton explains in *The Dark Side of Fat Loss*, this is akin to attempting to build a brick house on unstable foundations using unsound materials. No much wonder we fall apart! (Or gain weight or lack energy). The appropriate building blocks are critical.

Moreover, starve the body of fuel and it'll just retaliate by expending less. You'll have less energy, less muscle and a slower metabolism. None of which feels good. None of which creates lasting fat-loss. At some level you already know this. Starvation didn't work last time; it won't work this time either! It's the same idea with the those aiming to bulk up at the gym and the office workers just trying to get through their day: looking for that one trick to lose weight, build muscle or provide an energy boost isn't the answer.

Dieting on 1000 Calories a day does not nourish the body. Diet cola and energy drinks do not nourish the body. One special supplement or protein shake does not nourish the body. If you're ill or have bad skin or headaches or something more sinister, yep, drugs may temporarily alleviate your symptoms, but they do not nourish the body! We need a paradigm shift. We need to start by getting the body to function optimally. We need to start by getting our cells to run efficiently. We need to start with the right bricks! After all, an appropriately nourished body is unlikely to be a fat, sick and tired body - not for long anyway! Health is our default state!

So what provides the nourishment: the vitamins, minerals, enzymes, proteins, fats, carbohydrates and water that our cells need to run efficiently?

Real food.

REAL FOOD VS. INDUSTRIAL FOOD

"Where traditional cuisine is meant to satisfy, ...industrial food is meant to stimulate."
(David Kessler, author, The End of Overeating)

Eat 'real' food and eat enough to nourish the body. Sounds simple doesn't it? It kinda is. But here's the thing: many of us don't actually eat 'real' food any more. Times have changed and now, we mostly eat industrial food products. There is a difference between real food and industrial food. Food-manufacturing companies have shareholders to please - their goal is to increase profits. It's business. It is not about improving your health.

Our transition from 'real' food to industrial food is best summarised by Michael Pollan, in his excellent book *In Defence of Food*, in which he outlines five key nutritional changes:

1. We have moved from eating whole foods (foods close to how they appear in nature), to refined foods: stripping away much of the nutrients in the process and leaving us overstimulated and undernourished, full yet unsatisfied. I know you've experienced that!
2. We have moved from complexity to simplicity. At every level. "From the soil to the plate" as Pollan puts it. And we lose nourishment every step of the way.

3. We have moved from concerning ourselves with food quality: where our food comes from, what's actually in it, and how it's prepared, to obsessing over quantity: how many Calories, fat or carbs it contains, or how much we can eat.
4. We have moved from eating mostly leafy greens to eating mostly seeds. In particular, refined grains and rancid seed oils that can promote inflammation and illness in the body[12].
5. We have moved from food culture to food science. Where traditional wisdom and cooking practices were once passed down through the generations, we now get our advice from reductionist scientists who know better.

So what is 'real' food? Well, first of all, I prefer not to use labels around food. I don't want to promote any elitist attitudes about what we eat but, for the sake of simplicity, 'real food' is the term I'll use here.

By real food, I am referring to food made by nature – plants and animals. I am referring to 'whole' foods that don't require an ingredient list. Foods that can be prepared at home. Real food typically offers a whole lot of nourishment – vitamins, minerals and probably other things scientists either cannot measure or haven't discovered yet. Real food is the stuff that has kept the human race going for millions of years. Generally speaking, real food is *nutrient dense*: It contains a relatively high ratio of essential nutrients per mass of food. Nowadays, however, the majority of us consume products made by man that have lots of ingredients but not so many nutrients. We add preservatives and flavours and colours and substances that help create the right texture and 'mouthfeel', we get a whole lot of stimulation, but not so much nourishment. Not only do our cells not get the 'bricks' they need to run efficiently, some believe that this stimulation – food palatability and food reward – plays a role in overeating and obesity[13].

"The hedonic system influences how much you eat once you begin a meal – highly palatable food generally increases food intake by activating this system. Together, reward and hedonic circuitry in the brain determine in large part how often you eat, what you eat, and how much you eat, and this is influenced by the attributes of the food that's available."

(Stephan Guyenet, obesity researcher and blogger)[14]

Modern, processed food products are designed to be just that: palatable and rewarding. Food scientists know what attributes give food products these qualities. In *The End of*

Overeating, David Kessler explains how in recognising our innate desire for sweet, fat, and salty tastes, and by adding the right aroma, flavour, and texture, food companies are able to create what have been called *hyperpalatable* products. The combination of Calories, flavour hits, ease of eating, 'meltdown' and 'early hit' drive cravings, and Kessler also found that companies are able to add to their products almost any sensory effect they want us to feel! Products engineered in this way may provide stimulation way beyond what's normal for our brain and body (hence *hyper*-palatable) and disrupt normal appetite/satiety signals leading to overconsumption of these products[15]. The funny thing is, sometimes the companies will blatantly advertise the addictiveness! I even came across a breakfast cereal they actually named 'Krave®'! Am I the only one that sees something wrong with this?

"Rewarding foods are rewiring our brains. As they do, we become more sensitive to the cues that lead us to anticipate rewarding foods. [People] cannot control their responses to highly palatable foods because their brains have been changed by the foods they eat."

(David Kessler, author, The End of Overeating)

You probably know that Krave isn't the best breakfast choice, but even supposedly 'healthy' foods can offer more stimulation than nourishment. As we've had to become more health savvy, the food industry has responded by creating products with health claims. They've found ways to create low-Calorie and low-fat products by replacing traditional, nutrient dense fats like butter, with cheap alternatives like seed and vegetable oils. They've created sugar-free products laced with artificial sweeteners that make them even sweeter and just as stimulating as the more obvious junk foods. Yes, they might give us a brief energy boost, but we miss out on the nourishment we need so the energy boost is typically followed by a crash and more cravings. Whether they are marketed as 'healthy' or not, eating highly palatable industrial products can lead to overeating. Overeating can, in turn, lead to hormonal dysregulation like *insulin resistance*[16], which is associated with obesity and diabetes[17]. Hyperpalatable and high-energy industrial foods have also been suggested to play a role in *leptin resistance*[18]: a condition whereby the brain doesn't get the message that the body has sufficient fat stores[19]. So we might have more than enough fat, but our brain *thinks* we're too thin and acts accordingly – it drives us to eat more food and expend less energy so that our bodies can store yet more fat. Forget it: no amount of willpower is going to counter these powerful drives of the brain and body!

However, if we start by choosing nutrient dense, real foods, we nourish our body. We give it the bricks it needs to function properly. These foods – high-quality animal products, traditional fats (yes, that means real butter and other animal fats!), vegetables, fruit, and unprocessed grains – also tend to be more satiating, and less likely to be over consumed. These foods are much less likely to overstimulate the system and drive cravings. People tend not to binge wildly on mackerel or apples or asparagus. Without that overstimulation, we can receive the normal hormonal messages that cue us when to eat and, more importantly, when to stop eating. So rather than get hung up on the number of Calories, fat or carbs listed on the box, or swayed by the row of green ticks making cheerful health claims, look at the ingredients – if it's a giant list, if there are things on that list you need a chemistry degree to understand or that you cannot even pronounce, ask yourself if it's actually food? How much nourishment is it actually going to provide?

I'm not suggesting we should avoid all industrial food products. We don't want to turn eating into a religion, and such rigid behaviour tends to foster restrict-binge cycles (which I'll touch upon in the next section). But... successful eating plans have one thing in common: they cut out the majority of industrial products and focus on traditional, real foods, prepared at home. Not only does this strategy nourish our body, it usually helps us eat a more appropriate amount of food.

How do we recognise real food? There are always exceptions, but here are some questions to consider:

Is it made by man or by nature?
Was the food ever alive? ...where is that Special K tree?!
Would I require a factory to make this or could someone prepare it at home?
Does it have more than a few ingredients?
Do I understand the ingredients?
Does it have a shelf life?
Does it make health claims?
Would previous generations recognise this as food?
Have I seen this advertised on TV?!

FOOD BEHAVIOUR: THE *HOW* OF EATING

*The pleasure from eating...is more than the taste of the food and the feeling of a
full belly. Learn to enjoy the entire process – the hunger beforehand, the careful
preparation, setting an attractive table, chewing, breathing, smelling, tasting,
swallowing, and the feeling of lightness and energy after the meal. You can even
enjoy the full and easy elimination after it's digested. When you pay attention
to all elements of the process, you'll begin to appreciate simple meals.*

("Socrates" in The Way of the Peaceful Warrior by Dan Millman)

Have you ever noticed that so many experts out there, are great at advising us *what*
to do, but rarely actually offer any guidance on *how* to do it. I come across this a lot in
the fitness and nutrition industry. My Facebook news feed is full of 'tips' like "simply
swapping your crisps and chocolate for healthier options like fruit goes a long way".
Great insight. Thanks for that. If it were that easy, how come so many folks out there
don't have the energy and health they so badly desire? Oh, that's right, they're just lazy
gluttons.

I've struggled with binge eating. I know what it's like. Far from being an apparently,
robotically disciplined supertrainer like so many others out there, I get it. I also know
that amongst the overweight population are some of the most disciplined people
around. I've seen people commit to the daily pounding of the treadmill while enduring
diets that wouldn't nourish a butterfly. I understand why it's impossible to eat 'just
one', and why it's so hard to stop even though all you want to do is be slim/lean/toned.
I'm all too familiar with the dopamine rush when you decide to 'go for it': the surge
of excitement inevitably followed by heartache when the dust settles and you realise
you've done it again. ...Again! I've experienced the hopelessness and depression that
comes with cyclic self-sabotage. And yet I'm grateful for it. It has helped send me down
an incredible path of personal and professional growth. I've learned a lot about health,
about nutrition, about mindset and behaviour change. I've learned even more about
myself. Challenges really are gifts.

One insight I've learned is that we are *not* all lazy gluttons. It's not a *character flaw*; it's a
systems failure. We are not broken or lacking in willpower, we just need a better system,
a better strategy. As explained in Part One, mindset is critical. Finding our 'why' and
committing to a long-term approach of consistent, habit-based changes, one easy step

at a time, is the difference-maker that most of us don't respect. We write mindset off as unimportant and don't make the time to address it. Lets assume, however, that we're giving mindset the time and attention it deserves and we're now highly motivated to eat well. For the long haul. What are the key habits of food behaviour? What are the *hows*? What are our limiting factors when it comes to eating well?

From my experience of working with a wide range of clients, I believe it comes down to the *amount* of food we're eating, the *type* of food we're eating, or both.

If we're eating the wrong amounts, it could be because:

* We are not listening to our body
* We are listening to our body but the messages are faulty
* Mental-emotional cues encourage overeating (or undereating)

If it's the type of food we're eating that is the problem, it could be because:

* Those are the foods we have in our home. (Simple insight: you tend to eat what you have in your home!)
* We are disorganised so we eat whatever is available
* Our environment isn't supporting us.

Lets take a closer look.

RESTRAINED EATING

Our bodies are smart. They know when we need to eat and when we don't. Listen closely and they'll even indicate thirst or a preference for a certain type of food. But we don't listen. A common theme I see in those looking to lose weight is to ignore or suppress hunger cues. Lets repeat: to function properly our cells need nourishment. Starvation is not a sustainable weight loss strategy! Restricting Calories increases the output of stress hormones in the body.[20] Lets just say that's not a good thing! Hunger isn't designed to make us fat: it exists to keep us alive! Eat the food! Sometimes it's not Calories per se, but fat or sugar or something else that people blacklist. Recognise though, that we cannot willpower our way to good health. Restrained eating in general is associated with higher biomarkers of stress in the body[21,22]. It takes willpower to override our natural urges. Our willpower is limited, however, and it actually costs us energy – willpower uses up blood glucose[23]. Not only are "self-control failures...more likely when glucose is low"[24], but the use of willpower and resultant drop in blood sugar also adds to our stress load. Stress, in turn, makes us eat. It increases our appetite and, in particular, our cravings for sweet foods[25,26,27]. So we've used up our limited willpower and we've now got low blood sugar, reduced self-control, increased appetite and a craving for sweets. *And* we feel stressed. What could possibly go wrong?

> *"Focusing single-mindedly on not eating eventually pushes us to eat more. Feeling deprived only increases the reward value of food, and then usually gives way to indulgence, and often abandon. As desire evolves into need, we do exactly what we've tried so hard not to do – we eat that cream cake. And then we feel worse which makes us even more likely to be out of control."*
>
> (David Kessler, author, The End of Overeating)

Can you see how the very act of dieting (severely restricting Calories or restrained eating of any type) inevitably ends in failure? Typically, we then strengthen our resolve to eat *even stricter* and so the restrict-binge cycle is born. Indeed, rigid dieting is associated with both eating disorders and a higher body mass index when compared with a more flexible approach[28]. It just doesn't work. Obey your body. When it is crying out for food, eat! I like the idea of Zoe Harcombe, author of *The Harcombe Diet*, who suggests that we learn to treat ourselves, just not too much and not too often. Perhaps this sounds obvious, and it might not be an easy place to get to, but rather than being unnecessarily militant about our food choices and falling into reckless abandon whenever we do have a treat, this middle zone seems to be the place to aim for[29]. Better still, we could stop using labels like 'treats' and referring to ourselves or our food choices as 'good' or 'bad'. It's not a moral issue and indulging in dessert isn't a sin. If you must use labels, perhaps 'high/low quality' or 'nutritious/less nutritious' are more neutral and less emotionally charged ways to go. All this guilt we have around food benefits no one. There is no such thing as a 'good' or 'bad' food. Unless you've got an allergy or sensitivity to a specific food, there's not a single food that will make you overweight on its own. What matters is the overall context of the diet: not one food, but the big picture over a number of days, weeks or months.

For example, Sally might blame that "fattening" cheesecake for her weight gain, but her problem isn't that she ate some cheesecake, it's because she labelled cheesecake as "bad" and vowed never to eat that sort of stuff. So when she inevitably did 'break' her diet (and as we've just seen, it *is* inevitable), she went facedown in cheesecake. Knowing that cheesecake is a "banned" food and that she'd be back 'on the diet' tomorrow, she lost control. Subconsciously (or even consciously!) she made sure she got her fill of cheesecake today. It's a classic demonstration of the scarcity principle and the emotional arousal it generates:

> "The scarcity principle - that opportunities seem more valuable to us when their availability is limited."
>
> (Robert Cialdini, professor of psychology and author, Influence: The psychology of persuasion)

It was Sally's binge that shifted her average Calorie balance into weight-gain territory. It wasn't the cheesecake itself but the volume of cheesecake (and whatever else came with the binge). If Sally could let go of the idea that cheesecake was forbidden, she'd remove the scarcity element. She might then learn to be able to enjoy an occasional piece of cheesecake without the need to devour the lot. After all, she could have some more cheesecake tomorrow if she liked.

OVEREATING

The other side of the restrained eating coin is 'autopilot': when we do eat, we tend to eat on autopilot. We have got screen addiction: unable to drag ourselves away from our smartphones, computers or TV long enough to focus on our meal. Sometimes we eat while driving, sometimes we don't even sit down to eat. So what? Well, eating while distracted usually means we eat more. It's been shown that we eat slightly more in that moment (independent of dietary restraint), and even greater amounts later on[30]. Consider your own experiences: how many times have you finished a good meal only to be raking the cupboards for more food five minutes later? "What else can I have?" We've all munched through a bagful of sweets or crisps while watching TV only to reach the bottom of the bag and wonder where they've all gone. "I didn't eat *all* of those did I?" To eat appropriate amounts, we don't necessarily need to count Calories or weigh and measure everything we eat (do you really want to do that *forever*?); we need to pay attention. Sit down, slow down, take 15 minutes away from the screens and pay attention. Unless portion-sizes are fixed[31], people who eat more slowly tend to consume *less* food yet feel *more* satisfied than those who wolf down their food quickly[32]. An example of this is when we eat out, at a leisurely pace, in a restaurant which provides with modest portions of food. More often than not, even if we initially belittled the portion size, by the end of the meal we typically feel satisfied.

"When walking, walk. When eating, eat."

(Zen proverb)

Hunger also encourages us to eat too quickly[33]. If you're like me, there have probably been times when, in a famished state, you've raced through a big meal only to feel absolutely stuffed 20 minutes later when the satiety signals have caught up. Eating more slowly gives our brain the chance to recognise fullness before we overdo it. It also allows us the opportunity to be *mindful*, to actually enjoy our food – maybe even chew the stuff! (Which is pretty important for digestion). Obviously we want to avoid becoming too hungry in the first place. This can simply be achieved by eating regularly throughout the day and preparing high-quality food so that it is available to us when we need it.

CRAVINGS & MINDFUL EATING

When we eat mindfully: paying attention to, and obeying our body's signals, it becomes much easier to eat an appropriate amount of food. If we are truly eating mindfully (the vast majority of people don't even come close) and experience cravings, we have to look at the quality of our diet.

As explained earlier, industrial food products may disrupt the body's natural signalling. If we are eating too many hyperpalatable food products, we probably can't trust the signals our body gives us. In general, the more you eat cakes and crisps and cookies, the more you crave the stuff. It's self-reinforcing[34,35]. Moreover, if we are eating foods that fail to provide the nourishment our body needs we might find ourselves craving food even though we've just eaten. Calories might be abundant, but until the body receives the nourishment it requires, it's possible that it'll continue to send us signals to eat[36]. This theory explains why we experience the feeling of being full yet unsatisfied. The solution here is to focus on nourishment. Eat real food first. Since we don't want to go down that dark alley of dietary restraint, we won't consider less nutritious foods as 'banned' (Sally can still have her cheesecake in moderation), we just need to make sure we nourish our body with real food first. Funnily enough, when we do that, and do it mindfully, the appetite and desire for junk food diminishes.

If we experience cravings despite eating a nutritious diet, it would be prudent to listen to those cravings. There's wisdom there. Protein, fat and carbohydrates play important roles in the body and a craving for a sweet food, something fatty, or just a good old hunk of meat, could indicate that we are low on something that we need. For instance, when a client I was working with gave me a food diary revealing her very-low-fat diet, I guessed that she might have some serious cravings. I was right: the client went on to share that she couldn't keep real butter in her home because she'd eat the whole block in two days! Her body was screaming out for fat! I've made plenty of dietary mistakes in the past myself and after following a craving for raisins one day, I found myself devouring the entire 500g bag! Once I recovered from the upset stomach, the reason became obvious: my diet had been very low in carbohydrates and my body was demanding sugar. Clearly the solution lies not in periodic raisin binges but in listening to the clues and adjusting our diet accordingly. Carbohydrates and sugar aren't evil, and nor is fat! Believing that they are, and restricting them, only leads to problems.

> *"People who eat in response to hunger and satiety cues, have unconditional permission to eat, and cope with feelings without food, [and] are less likely to engage in eating behaviors that lead to weight gain."*
>
> *(Madden et al, 2012[37])*

This concept of *intuitive eating* can take some practice and being mindful of our body's signals is important[38], but I believe that, for most, it's a wiser, more sustainable option than attempting to scientifically determine our exact nutritional requirements and then weigh and measure everything that crosses our lips. Intuitive eating in general is associated with an increase in the enjoyment and pleasure of food, lower body mass index, and fewer dieting behaviours and food anxieties[39,40]. There is also a correlation with other positive health markers such as lower triglycerides, higher HDL cholesterol and reduced cardiovascular risk[41].

That being said, tracking Calories and macronutrients (protein, fat and carbohydrates) does have its place. It allows us see if we're in the ballpark as regards to quantity of food we're eating, and it can be a useful strategy to adopt from time to time. For certain people – such as weight-class athletes and physique competitors – it may even be necessary. However, it can also be a burden and, for some people, it can promote obsessive behaviour. It can distract us from tuning into our bodies: blindly following a nutrition plan without listening to your own body and paying attention to how you feel is likely to lead to frustration. Take responsibility and find out what works for you. Rather than fight your natural urges, roll with them: start with real food, be self-compassionate and give your body what it needs. Forget the dogma and nutrition tribalism.

MENTAL-EMOTIONAL INFLUENCES

Before we discuss the challenges around eating the right *type* of foods, it's important to recognise that our motivation to eat is not purely physiological. Overeating and undereating can be triggered by mental-emotional factors too. Stress, tiredness and depression are perhaps the most obvious triggers, but there are others. For me, overeating can be a "shadow activity", a way of avoiding doing what's important. It's also an escape from boredom. It's a classic manifestation of the 'Resistance' brilliantly described by Steven Pressfield in his books *The War of Art* and *Turning Pro* (tip: read those books!). I'm sure many can relate to the mystical draw of the frequent 'kitchen break' when you're at a loose end or have some work that you're procrastinating on. That's Resistance.

Curiously, free food seems to hold some hidden power too. I've found myself making choices I wouldn't normally dream of making if I was actually buying the stuff in a shop or restaurant – just because it's there and it's free. Can you relate to the following scenarios?

* You might not feel like having a cookie and, in that moment you certainly wouldn't go out of your way to buy one, but because they've been laid out next to the teas and coffees you help yourself to two or three.

* Someone's retiring so there's a big box of chocolates in the office. You spend all day grazing on them. It's ok, it's a one-off, it's Jim's last day after all. But next week is Suzie's birthday, the week after that John is celebrating becoming a father and we *always* have muffins on a Friday.

* The buffet is still open and there are still piles of food. You're not hungry, you wouldn't *pay* for another course, but there you are loading up your plate once again. It'd be a shame to waste it, right?

For many people, when food is free, the game changes.

Another trigger is specific locations with which we associate with eating, or eating particular foods. I'm pretty sure not *everyone* at the cinema is hungry. Many people don't even enjoy cinema food! As with free food, it's just automatic: cinema = snacks. My dad always had sweets and treats in his home when I was younger and even now

I find it hard to break the association with eating something every time I visit him – regardless of my physical appetite! Maybe it's a particular shop that you associate with buying a treat, or maybe you associate visiting your Grandparents with eating chocolate biscuits. Maybe Friday night by default equals takeaway night!

Whether it's stress, free food, autopilot routines we run in certain situations, or something else altogether, the first step in eradicating this type of overeating or undereating is awareness. By all means enjoy a snack at the movies and indulge yourself on Jim's retirement, just do it by choice, not by pre-programmed routine. Habit has been shown to one of the most powerful predictors of eating behaviour[42], so if behaviours like these are a limiting factor in your diet, take the time to identify them. If you regret eating so much, get curious – what triggered that? Keep a journal and look for patterns in your eating behaviour. To alter a habit, you need a contingency plan, what are you going to do instead?

OUR FOOD ENVIRONMENT

Our environment shapes so many of our choices in life, and food is no exception. So in addressing the *type* of foods we eat, the first step is to build an environment that supports us. If we tend to eat what's available, it's wise to keep our homes stocked with real food and reduce the number food products that offer more stimulation than nourishment. Review the real food questions – if you find yourself snacking on sweets and crisps every night, maybe you should stop keeping them in your home. Again, they are not banned; it's just smart not to live with temptation in the cupboards while trying to change a habit. If it's there, you know you're going to eat it – most likely when you least need it, and as part of some unconscious routine you've developed. Please don't tell me you need stacks of junk food at home for the kids or for guests. It doesn't do them any good either! It's curious to me that many pet owners will only feed their dogs the highest quality foods. "Don't give him that", they say, "it's poisonous to dogs". Yet we are quite happy to feed our children and ourselves a diet based around poor quality food products on a daily basis. Do we really respect the dog's health more than that of our children or our selves? Once we've cleared out the low-quality stuff, the next step is to go shopping and stock up on real food. Get some eggs, meat, fish, vegetables and fruits. Grab some saturated fat for cooking with (coconut oil, butter, ghee, goose fat or duck fat are good choices). A variety of herbs and spices are also a valuable addition.

Everybody is busy nowadays. We actually brag about how busy we are. If we are that busy, it's a good idea to know a few recipes we can throw together with minimum fuss. Good food can be prepared quickly and easily and there are infinite recipe resources online to support every style of eating. Find a few quick and easy recipes that suit you. When time permits, you can experiment a little more. Make a list of some simple recipes and snacks you can take with you to work or if you're travelling. A lot of our poorer food choices are made as a result of availability: low-quality food is everywhere! Given the choice many of us would opt for a hearty, home-cooked meal ahead of some pre-packaged store-bought stuff, but we don't give ourselves that choice. Real food feels better; it's just not as widely available or convenient. This is where a little preparation helps. Again, it's not a character flaw; it's a systems failure, and more often than not, the issue people have isn't actually with the food itself; the issue is with creating a routine, a system, an *environment*, that supports helpful eating.

We like to think we make our own decisions but we're more susceptible to subtle environmental influences than we'll ever believe (or admit to!). In *Mindless Eating*, Brian Wansink details several studies that demonstrate this influence, such as one in which chocolates were given to receptionists. Experimenters had the chocolates placed a glass dish on the receptionist's desk. As anticipated, the receptionists ate the chocolates. In another setting, the glass dish was substituted for an opaque dish and the experimenters noticed that when the chocolates were not clearly visible, the receptionists ate fewer of them. When the chocolates were moved out of sight altogether – to the desk drawer – even fewer were consumed. The final setting saw the chocolates placed not just out of sight, but a few metres away, making them less available, and – you guessed it – the receptionists ate fewer still. It's important to note that in each setting the receptionists had not been asked to resist the chocolates; on the contrary, they'd been given them as gifts! The number of chocolates consumed was determined not by hunger or stress or even habit, but by the set-up of the environment.

"People's ability to identify the factors that influence their behavior is surprisingly poor."
(Goldstein, Martin & Cialdini, Yes: 50 Secrets from the science of persuasion)

A similar study took place in a cinema where everybody was given free popcorn. Free, two-week-old, stale popcorn! Half of the audience received a large box, the other half a small box. Despite the popcorn being just as undesirable to both groups, those with the bigger boxes ate more. The lesson: when eating from a bigger container, we subconsciously assume a larger portion size. So if you buy stuff in bulk, it might be helpful to break it up into lots of smaller containers to be stored separately. Similar experiments have been done with sweets. If I were to give you a bag of 100 sweets, you would likely eat more sweets than if I gave you the same 100 sweets divided into in ten bags of ten. People shake their heads, "nope, that kind of stuff doesn't influence me", but the studies repeatedly show otherwise. (This is why we are increasingly sold large 'share bags' of sweets and crisps or 'twinpacks' of chocolate. By putting several portions in one package, the companies know we'll eat more ...and buy more! It's better value after all, right?). Wansink also describes how smaller plates have been shown to help reduce overconsumption. It's like one of those optical illusions: food presented on a large plate looks substantially less than the same quantity placed on a smaller plate. So with bigger plates, we mindlessly eat more than we need. Oh, and Wansink reports that nowadays we generally use much bigger dinner plates!

By making minor tweaks to our environment – making low-quality foods less available, keeping food out of sight, serving from smaller containers onto smaller plates – Wansink argues that we can avoid overconsumption without even trying. On the other hand, for those who need to eat more, the opposite can be done: leave food in sight, pour from large containers and serve on big plates!

PARAMETERS

The reason it's easier to control our behaviours (and Calories) when 'on a diet' is because of the diet's *parameters*. Parameters – rules and guidelines – make things black and white. They take the decision-making away from us so there's no internal debate. The problem is that the parameters typically involve some form of restrained eating or unnecessarily rigid rules that prove to be completely unsustainable in the long run. So we fail. It's the very reason people go *on* a diet. It's seen as something we do short-term. 'Diet', however, should not be a verb, but a noun. It is not something we *do*, it is something that *is*: it's just how we eat. It's our food philosophy. We can still benefit from parameters; we just need to set our guidelines around the sustainable fundamentals of good nutrition. From those guidelines, we build our habits in the manner described in Part One: one easy step at a time.

So, in summary, the fundamentals of happy food behaviour are:

Nourishment
- Eat for nourishment rather than for weight loss or an energy boost.
- Eat real food first and avoid restrained eating.

Mindfulness
- Eat slowly and chew your food.
- Eat undistracted – turn off the screens!
- Consider mental-emotional cues and get curious about your triggers.

Intuitive Eating
- Listen to and obey hunger and satiety signals.
- Pay attention to cravings – what is your body telling you?
- Eat regularly to manage hunger.

Environment
- Remove low-quality foods from your home.
- Stock your home with real food.
- Find a few satisfying recipes you can prepare with ease.
- List some simple, real food snacks and be prepared.
- Keep food out of sight (or in sight if undereating is your limiting factor!)
- Use smaller containers and plates (or larger if undereating is your limiting factor!).

NON-FOOD NOURISHMENT

SLEEP

It's easy to forget that as important as nutrition is, it's not the complete picture when it comes to optimising our energy. One of the most crucial and commonly overlooked health components is sleep. Sleep helps to regulate our hormones – especially those involved in controlling our appetite[43,44,45,46]. When we don't sleep, our hormones can become a little messed up, leading us to spontaneously consume more food[47]. There go those faulty messages again.

While we have to be careful in how we interpret scientific studies[‡], restricted sleep has been repeatedly associated with blood sugar problems and is implicated as a risk factor for diabetes[48,49], and obesity[50,51], – indeed, just a single night of sleep loss can induce the insulin resistance mentioned above[52]. Short sleep duration is also linked with higher levels of inflammation in the body[53,54], (think pain and the onset of illness - not good!). It affects our brain[55], memory[56], attention[57], perhaps even our happiness in general. Again, lets not confuse correlation with causation, but there is even a relationship between chronic sleep problems and greater risk for "suicidality"[58].

In our busy lives, it's easily forgotten: sleep matters. Here are some strategies for improving our sleep:

1. Control the light

This is a game-changer. Our bodies are naturally tuned to light and darkness. When it's dark we should go to sleep – when the sun brings light, we wake. Anyone who has been camping knows this. You also know that it's easier to get up early and stay up late in the summer compared with the dark winters.

* Sleep in a pitch-black room: invest in a blackout blind or blackout curtains (or both!).
* Keep technology out of the bedroom: the flashing lights do nothing to help (nor does the distraction).
* Try using a wake-up light alarm clock: The light gradually dims at night and gradually lights up in the morning – how it's meant to be!
* Turn off the screens at least 15 minutes before bed and dim the lights if possible - this includes smartphones, TVs, computers, and portable devices. Turn it all off!

---

‡ It's difficult to do a properly controlled sleep study with more than just a few participants so most of the research is on only small groups or relies on heavily on associations (remember correlation does not necessarily equal causation - umbrellas don't cause rain!).

2. Form routines

In the same way athletes use pre-competition routines to get them fired up, a bedtime routine can help prepare our mind and body for sleep.

- Create a consistent sleep cycle: where possible, get up and go to bed the same time every day. Our body likes routine and it will be much easier to get up in the mornings.
- Reserve the bedroom for sleeping (and intimate activities): avoid doing work or other leisure activities in the bedroom. We want to associate being in there with relaxing and sleeping. Why do you need a TV in there?
- Adopt a bedtime routine: wind down in a consistent way. This includes dimming the lights and turning off the screens. Include journaling, a night-time drink or going for a walk in the evening. These can all relax mind and body.

3. Calm down & switch off

Sometimes it can be hard to switch off the mind. Try these:

- Avoid stimulants in the afternoon/evening: caffeine in particular can keep us feeling wired and disrupt sleep. For some people exercise late in the day can do the same.
- Try a night-time drink: warm milk has historically worked for some. Try the 'night time' tea by
  Pukka Teas or a magnesium drink like Natural Calm.
- Journal your thoughts: if you struggle with thoughts racing around your head at night, a useful strategy is to journal. Empty your mind by downloading all those thoughts onto paper. It helps ...and not just your sleep.

NATURE

Another overlooked tool in enhancing our energy and overall wellbeing is interacting with nature. The benefits of interacting with nature are clear: science suggests that time in nature improves cognitive function[59] and has restorative[60] and stress-reducing[61] qualities. It enhances mood and memory – in both healthy and depressed[62] groups and is seen as a key promoter of health and wellbeing[63,64]. Lets be honest, who doesn't feel better after a forest walk or a stroll along the beach? Getting out in nature is also likely to mean more exposure to the sunlight that we depend on heavily for vitamin D. Vitamin D deficiency is said to be one of the most common medical conditions worldwide[65] and is linked to many chronic diseases including autoimmune diseases, infectious diseases, cardiovascular disease and deadly cancers[66]. Of course getting sunburnt is a bad idea, but sensible sun exposure plays an important role in our overall health. If you live in a climate like the one here in the north-east of Scotland, those few sunny days are precious! Get outside!

COMMUNITY

Our relationships with others also play an important role in our energy and general wellbeing. It has been suggested that as humans we have a basic need to belong[67], to have a sense of community with others, and that a lack of such attachment is detrimental to our health and longevity[68,69]. Community with others can take a variety of forms: ties to family, neighbours, work-related communities and other groups are related our overall life satisfaction and happiness – both directly and by impacting our health[70,71].

Of course, just joining any old group of people might not be the best thing for our energy. You know as well as I do that there are people who are a better influence on your life than others. Some people lift us up: they encourage the best parts of us and we feel energised by their mere presence. Then there are those 'energy vampires' who seemingly suck every drop of life out of us. Kryptonite. (It has even been suggested that obesity can spread through social ties![72]).

> *"Stop taking advice from broke, unhappy people."*
> *(David Wood, business leader, coach and podcaster: The Kick-Ass Life Show)*

Personal development gurus have long told us that we become our peers: those we hang out with most. The trick is, therefore, to surround ourselves with the type of people who energise us. I'm not suggesting we need to abruptly disown our family and break all of our friendships but it would be helpful to develop an awareness of which relationships are positive and which are less so. We have to protect our energy!

Today's information age offers an unparalleled opportunity to connect with great people. Never before have we had such easy access to some of the best minds on the planet – in any field. Books, music, podcasts, online videos and courses all provide incredible opportunities to expose ourselves to new ideas and surround ourselves with those who can enhance our lives. Through social media, it has also become increasingly easy to actually connect with great people and to join communities or 'mastermind groups' with like-minded individuals. I've done this myself and have been able to meet in person and study under some truly inspiring leaders in my field. In my opinion, finding an appropriate role model, coach or mentor is one of the best things you can do for your life. (And, hey, if you've read this far, why not come connect with me on Facebook.com/AKRMike or Twitter @AKRConditioning. I'm certainly no guru, but I would love to hear what you think of the book. I'd love to hear what habits and goals you're working on).

Of course online connections and community aren't quite the same as human contact, and while meeting a role model can be a buzz, it's helpful if we can develop mutually positive relationships with people in our everyday lives. Perhaps there is a club or group you can join — uplifting people tend to be the proactive type, so trying new hobbies and experiencing new things represents a great way to find an energising community. Yep, stepping into new environments can be scary, it always is when you leave a comfort zone, but that fear is just The Chimp talking anyway!

> *"Do the thing you fear, and the death of fear is certain."*
> *(Ralph Waldo Emerson, essayist, lecturer, and poet)*

MOVEMENT
The final piece I want to discuss is movement. There's a lot to say — so much in fact that I'm giving it it's own section. See you in part 3...

PART TWO SUMMARY

* Food is confusing because as individuals we have different requirements.
* The first goal of nutrition should be to nourish our body.
* In general, real food offers more nourishment whereas industrial food offers more stimulation.
* Restrained eating does not work.
* Mindfulness is a key component of healthy eating behaviour.
* Intuitive eating is associated with positive diet and health behaviours.
* Mental-emotional factors influence our food choices.
* Habit is one of the most powerful predictors of eating behaviour.
* By tweaking our food environment, we can alter our eating behaviour.
* Setting parameters can help guide our food behaviour.
* Sleep has a profound impact on our appetite, health and wellbeing.
* Time in nature is a key promoter of health and wellbeing.
* As humans, we have a basic need to for social connection.
* Our social ties can enhance or destroy our energy.
* We have opportunities to connect inspiring people and mentors.

PART THREE >

Exercise

Exercise. It's another word that means different things to different people. The word itself has pretty powerful connotations: it can conjure up images of drudgery and torture, or joyful play. It can be our mortal enemy or our best friend. For me – as ever – it comes down to perception: what's the purpose of exercise?

MOVEMENT

The problem many people get themselves into is viewing exercise only as a means of burning Calories, a tool for weight-loss. This viewpoint has a couple of major flaws. Firstly, it takes an awful lot of exercise to burn Calories relative to what's in food. We've all seen those tables that show just how much jogging is needed to 'burn off' last night's slice of pizza or chocolate bar (answer: a lot!). For good reason "you cannot out-train a bad diet" has become a mantra for personal trainers everywhere. In diet vs. exercise, diet always wins: Calories can be consumed much more readily and in greater abundance than they can be burned in an exercise session. Unfortunately, this realisation is what often leads people into the pitfall of dietary restriction, malnourishment and starvation discussed in Part Two. "If I can't burn all those Calories off, I'll just eat less", is the thinking. This thinking doesn't help. Yes, Calories matter. But so does breathing – and we don't need to regulate our breath nor consciously force breath in and out of the body. Exercise isn't just about how many Calories we can burn today combined with how much starvation we can endure. Moreover, the types of exercise people gravitate to for their Calorie-burning fix tend – for the most part – to be mind-numbing hours spent chugging along on the cross-trainer or treadmill, day after day after day. Sure it can be ok to begin with, but let's be honest, it's not a lot of fun and it doesn't produce great results.

"Motion is life."
(Hippocrates, Greek physician)

Does that mean exercise is a waste of time? No. When it comes to good energy, exercise - *movement*! - is essential. Whoever we are, wherever we are, we need to move. Movement is a requisite for good energy. In fact it's a requisite for life: only things that are dead don't move. Although our heart functions like a pump, our body still relies on physical movement to help in the transportation of substances around our body. Movement keeps things moving: helpful substances are brought in and waste products tidied out more efficiently. Muscles and connective tissues are kept supple and slide smoothly over one another. We function better.

So the first purpose of exercise is to move, and to move well. I've had my share of injures and I know as well as you do that painful, stiff or restricted movement can be calamitous for our energy – both physically and mentally – even if we do look lean and athletic. It's just a shame that so many people nowadays move so poorly that they've no concept of how uplifting free and easy movement can be. When done well, physical movement feels fantastic. Moreover, when we move our body, we also move our mind, and a better mood and mental state is our reward. Change your *physiology* and you change your *psychology*. Try it now: put a ridiculous smile on your face and dance around the room a little. You'll feel better. That's that increased blood flow.

> *"Your tissues are designed to be 110 years old. You just have to know what the stable, tissue-saving, catastrophe-avoiding positions are. And, you have to practice them. A lot."*
>
> *(Dr. Kelly Starett, physical therapist, coach & author, Becoming a Supple Leopard)*

Like so many other deteriorations in our health, restricted movement is seen as a 'normal' result of ageing. Lets not confuse what's *common* with what's *normal* for the human body. Restricted movement is a result of less movement. It's a cliché but it really is a case of 'use it or lose it', and since the vast majority of us spend our lives sitting on our backsides, we lose it. It's not ageing that makes our muscles and joints stiff and sore, it's neglect. When we do move, we do so with a focus on burning those Calories in a bid to look good, all the while forgetting that supple, effortless movement is one of the most beautiful sights there is (just picture your favourite athlete in action - or a dancer or gymnast[H]). As a result, we choose repetitive, limited range exercises that have the potential to destroy our body if we are not already functioning well.

[H] For some serious movement inspiration check out 'Ido Portal' on YouTube)

"You can lift with a rounded back, run like crap, and sit at your computer with your neck and shoulders rounded for a long time ... until you can't. That's when your body offers up some hard truths – that you've been moving incorrectly or that you've been hanging out in bad positions. And it doesn't just whisper in your ear – it crams the message down your throat by zapping your ability to generate force and opening the floodgates to pain."

(Dr. Kelly Starett, physical therapist, coach & author, Becoming a Supple Leopard)

Running hundreds of miles with poor movement, or deadlifting massive amounts of weight with faulty mechanics will inevitably cause stress, wear out our bodies and crush our energy. And that's not to mention the perils of sitting! Forget Calories, quality movement comes first. Move!

What is quality movement? It is taking our joints through a full range of motion and being able to smoothly perform the basic, physical tasks of the human animal: squatting, bending, lunging, pushing, pulling, twisting, and locomotion (walking-jogging-running) – without pain. Quality movement feels good and we're able to navigate life better. Movement is a gift! While a thorough examination of movement quality is beyond the scope of this book**, physical therapist and author, Gray Cook, in his book, *Movement*, identifies 5 basic principles we should be aware of:

1. Basic bodyweight movements should not produce pain.

If we experience pain, we should address it. Too many of us get injured and address only the symptom. We strap up the knee and get on with it, forgetting to consider what actually *caused* the injury. Without addressing the cause (perhaps mobility/stability issues or muscle imbalances), it's likely that the injury, or another, will reappear.

We also love to ignore the injury and look instead for a workaround – something to get us through the workout – like an exercise modification or a strapping. In doing this we're looking for a fitness solution to what is a medical problem. If my clients tell me they have pain in a movement, it is outwith my scope of practice to diagnose or treat it. I tell them – and you – to seek out a medical professional. We're prone to this behaviour outside the exercise context too – people look for something to mask the symptom (painkillers, medications, avoiding particular activities), rather than addressing the cause.

** Check out *Becoming a Supple Leopard* by Dr. Kelly Starett or *Athletic Body in Balance* by Gray Cook for a more detailed guide to improving your movement quality.

2. Restricted movement, even if pain-free, can increase injury risk and lead to secondary problems.

Even if there's no pain at present, if you are tight, stiff and restricted in basic movements, you may well be heading toward future problems. I do a basic movement screen with all new clients and have found that movement limitations are fairy common – especially in office workers who sit all day long. I also see it in those who've spent years participating in one particular sport or fitness pursuit and have neglected mobility work in their training (footballers and runners being prime examples).

You might not have noticed the limitation, as our body will always find a way to get the job done: we'll compensate and substitute where necessary even if it means wearing out joints by using them improperly. You may need the help of a professional, or you may just need to practice the movement more. Either way, focus on improving the movement.

3. Basic movements involving the body's left and right sides should be mostly symmetrical.

Remember we're talking movement here. Of course one side might be more coordinated or skilful than the other. When it comes to movement, however, we should have a good degree of symmetry. I often hear people explaining that their tight calf or sore shoulder, for instance, is down to 'doing too much' that week. I always ask: if both sides did the same work, why is it that only the right side is sore? It sounds like there might be an imbalance somewhere and if you are training for something repetitive like a marathon or a kettlebell sport event involving ten minutes of jerks (an overhead pressing exercise), this imbalance could limit your performance and lead to injury.

4. Basic movement skills should come before performance-based exercise.

If you can't keep your spine straight while bending, it's probably not the best idea to go for that heavy deadlift. Or as renowned movement teacher, Ido Portal, says, *"If you cannot move your body and control it...then what business do you have moving other objects outside of you – if you cannot control your own self"*[73]. This applies not only to weightlifting, but any form of exercise.

5. Basic movement skills should come before more complex movements.

This one is a problem for your average gym buff *and* personal trainers. In order to keep sessions exciting, to be seen at the cutting edge, trainers love to give fancy new exercises to their clients. But there's no point in doing that 'one-leg-Bosu-squat-with-an-off-set-kettlebell-with-your-eyes-closed', if you've yet to master the bodyweight squat or the bodyweight pistol squat. Simplicity before complexity.

I'll leave it to Gray Cook to summarise:

"Pain produced by movement should be reported, managed, diagnosed and treated by a medical professional.

Manage movement pattern limitations and asymmetries – mobility and stability problems – before applying a significant volume of fitness, performance and sports training."

(Gray Cook, author, Movement)

PERFORMANCE

When we see exercise through performance rather than solely a means of emptying our fuel tank, we make it more interesting. Rather than focussing on weight-loss (which tends to be more influenced by diet and lifestyle anyway), I encourage my clients to choose a *performance goal*. Having a self-chosen performance goal can be highly motivating: it enables us to capture that sense of autonomy which I discussed in Part One and which is so critical for lasting motivation.

By continually working to fine-tune our performance – especially with a skill-based activity – we give ourselves the opportunity to become lost in a state of deep practice: that commitment to mastery I discussed in Part One. I've seen this over and over again as clients get excited about their journey to achieve core competences like a pull-up or push-up. I've seen people eager work on their kettlebell technique at every available opportunity and, in my own exercise programme, I've found myself engaged for months in a project to mastering a one-arm, one-leg push-up. Every workout was a chance to get better. Every step forward was positive reinforcement and an increase in my self-efficacy. It's harder to achieve that if you're just burning Calories. Strength is a practice.

Recall that the third aspect of the new approach to motivation is purpose – our why. Rather than the somewhat abstract notion of weight-loss, a performance goal is easier to tie to something more meaningful. This could be in an athletic context or simply performance in your everyday life. Does your body function well enough to get you through your typical routine? Can you climb the stairs and carry the shopping without fuss? Do you have the energy to play with the kids? Will you in the future? Or are you slowly drifting down that fun path of limited function, creaky fragility and eventual dependency on others? Ageing doesn't have to be like that. What if today wasn't a typical day? What if you found yourself in some sort of emergency situation today, how would your body fare? Could you literally run for your life – or someone else's – if you had to? Could you jump or pull your bodyweight up and out of window in a burning building? Could you lift a small child or dear friend and carry them to safety? Or are you the person whose poor physical condition puts the lives of others in jeopardy? Could your inability to perform physically cost someone else his or her life? How's that for purpose? Is all that moderate cardio and Calorie burning really improving your athleticism, your performance in life?

The great thing is that with our performance goal fuelling our motivation, exercise begins to feel a lot more like play than it does a chore. It's more inspiration than obligation. The perspiration is still there – we're still burning Calories – so over time we change the way our body looks anyway!

FUN

Another often forgotten aspect of exercise is fun. Exercise can be fun. It's heart-breaking to see so many joggers trudging along out there looking miserable but dutifully putting in their miles in the cold, in the dark, in the wind and horizontal rain that are synonymous with the winter here in Scotland (sometimes spring, summer and autumn aren't much better!). I have nothing against running itself, in fact I considered doing my city's 10k this year (a nice performance goal) but with the weather being what it was, there were few days I felt I'd actually enjoy running outside. So I didn't. There are other ways to move. There are other ways to be healthy. There are other ways to have fun.

Exercise can be play. Sure, you might not enjoy every workout, but it doesn't need to be the sadomasochistic beatdown that has become so popular nowadays. Harder, tougher, faster, longer. 'Ultra' this and 'extreme' that. "Go hard or go home". If you enjoy it, cool, but you don't have to kill yourself in a 6 am spin class every morning. It doesn't need to be a chore. One of my clients has a hoodie that reads: 'Train insane or remain the same.' It's a nice mantra – catchy – and I'm all for hard work. I'm not sure it's true though. We don't need to crush ourselves in order to improve. We must remember that exercise is a stress on the body and during exercise we're actually breaking our tissues down. It's during our recovery – with adequate rest, sleep and good nutrition – that we change and improve in response to the stimulus of exercise. If we're constantly beating ourselves up in the gym, when does our body get the chance to adapt and grow stronger?

"Stressed out? Forget about getting a healthy adaptation response to that crushingly difficult workout – you will simply get crushed."

(Dr. Kelly Starett, physical therapist, coach & author, Becoming a Supple Leopard)

Besides, say like most, we're *already* broken down. Say we're *already* low on energy. If we're already tired, unhealthy, inflamed, under chronic stress, and/or emotionally worn out, is forcing ourselves through that workout really going to help? Probably not, and nor is panicking or becoming guilt-ridden over the odd missed session. Stop beating yourself up and just go have some fun. Do something you actually enjoy. It could be dancing, climbing, games and sports, or just picking up heavy stuff. Get outside. Connect with friends. Move your body.

EFFECTIVENESS

"Working hard and working long are not the same. And neither one means working effectively."

(Alwyn Cosgrove, fitness coach, author & gym owner)

Aside from choosing exercises that aren't much fun, the majority of people I see in gyms aren't doing what's effective either. Pick any 'big-box' gym and you'll see the same faces doing the same thing at the same time every day: they even use the same machine. In one gym I worked at you could have blindfolded me and I'd still have been able to tell you who was in, what they were doing, and where. 'Cross trainer lady' on the machine second from the end. She'll do 30 minutes. 'Leg press guy' up the back. The guy in the vest who spends most of his time doing crunches. The woman with the blue top jogging on the treadmill nearest the wall. Are they improving the way they look, feel and perform? It's unlikely. Come back a year later and they'll look exactly the same. Or they'll have vanished altogether only to return again in January ...with the same old routine! The sad fact is that most of the people in the gym aren't getting results. This especially sad for me since my role is to help people improve. Clearly we need to do a better job of getting the message out!

When we realise that we are not making progress, we have two options: give up, or change something. Giving up is never the answer and, happily, many people do opt to make a change. The problem lies in the typical changes we make. The usual first step is to simply do more. 30 minutes on the treadmill three times per week didn't work so we'll do 40 minutes. In training speak, this is called increasing the *duration*. If that doesn't work, we might increase the *frequency* - we'll resolve to train more often. If those three classes each week aren't helping, lets up it to five or six. That *might* help; moving more often is good and we're burning more Calories after all. But there are plenty of folks training every day who still don't have the results they crave. And where does it end?

There was a girl in a gym I worked in whom we'll call Jill. Jill started off with the typical cross-trainer workout. First she increased the time she exercised each session. It wasn't long though before I noticed Jill doing 'double-sessions'. She'd do 45 minutes on the cross-trainer in the morning, then another 45 minutes in the afternoon. But Jill still wasn't happy with her results. Worse, she seemed to have become a 'cardio-junkie'. Jill found that if she missed a session all of those Calories didn't get burned and she would gain weight! She *had* to do it! Moreover, as her body adapted, she got more efficient at her routine. So Jill became dependent on working out more and more just to stay more or less the same! Remember, we adapt during recovery. Not only does continually doing more and more, more often, leave little room for recovery, it is totally unsustainable!

If we've not yet given up hope, some of us might come to the realisation that it's not just about duration and frequency and we'll decide to increase the *intensity*. We'll leave our comfort zone and we'll work harder. We'll perform more work in the same period of time (or in much less time). This might help too. Higher intensity exercise has been shown to be superior to moderate exercise for improving aerobic capacity[74,75] and promoting fat loss[76,77,78] in a variety of groups including high risk groups like those with heart disease[79] and heart failure,[80] and conditions such as rheumatoid arthritis[81]. More vigorous exercise is even associated with greater longevity[82]. In those who are already highly trained, high-intensity interval training may well be the *only* way to further increase endurance performance[83]. Getting the intensity right means creating a stimulus for our body to adapt to. Our body is effectively saying, "WHOA! That was harder than usual, I'd better get stronger so I'm ready for next time!" We have to continually expose our body to a greater challenge than before. This concept is known as *progressive overload* and while many use duration, volume (total amount of exercise) and frequency to create an overload, increasing the intensity tends to be low on our list - even though it allows us be more efficient with our time. It also helps us avoid wrecking our body by simply doing way too much. An example would be if Jill replaced some of her high volume, moderate-intensity, 45-minute cross-trainer sessions with a few sprint sessions comprising of just 5-10 minutes of high-intensity interval training. Happily this is exactly what Jill did, and by also adding some strength training, she was able to break her cardio dependency and actually start seeing some results – not to mention saving an incredible amount of time!

Aside from altering the intensity, this change in Jill's programme – particularly with the addition of strength training – did something else really important. It made Jill's training more *effective*. Unfortunately, effectiveness is something that most recreational exercisers and gym goers never actually consider. We can work as long, as often, even as *hard* as we want, but if our training methodology – the exercises we do or the programme we follow – isn't *effective*, then we'll get limited results at best, and zero results, injuries and become disillusioned at worst. Do this long enough and it can be pretty damaging to our self-esteem and self-efficacy. Our failure in the health and fitness realm can easily spread into the rest of our life. There are countless people who've spent a lifetime battling demons around their bodyweight or body image. Years of effort and no reward. Never mind energy, it can destroy our whole identity.

We need to train smarter. Few people would prepare for a bodybuilding contest by running marathons. Few would improve their 10k time by focussing most of their efforts on biceps curls. That would be ridiculous! It's just not effective. Ok, I've chosen a couple of absurd examples and maybe you think my point is an obvious one. It's not. As a personal trainer, I'm in the gym almost every day and I see how most people exercise. I also have a good idea of what their goal is. My conclusion is this: most of us don't train effectively. If you're frustrated with your results, you either need a little more patience (chopping and changing programmes every two weeks doesn't help!), or, as I said at the top of this section, you need to make a change. When making that change, we need to be smart. As one of the best in the business, Alwyn Cosgrove, says, *"More is not better, better is better".*

Effectiveness first. Intensity second. Frequency third. Volume last.[84]

EFFECTIVE TRAINING FOR FAT LOSS

So what does effective training look like? Clearly, it would be impractical for me to discuss effective training for every possible health and fitness outcome. Instead, I'll focus on effective training for the most common goal: fat loss.

UNDERSTANDING METABOLISM

When the goal is fat loss, Calories matter. Just maybe not in the way we've been led to believe. First we must understand a little about metabolism. The image below roughly represents the breakdown of Calories we burn in a day.

Energy expenditure

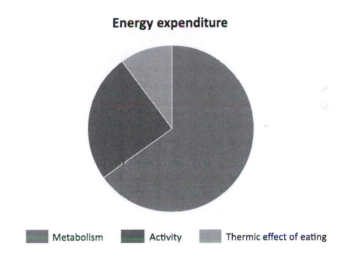

Metabolism   Activity   Thermic effect of eating

Around 60-70% of the total Calories we burn each day are the energy used for our *basal metabolic rate* – what we generally refer to as our metabolism. This is the energy the body uses for basic functioning. More than just Calories though, our metabolism is the sum of all cellular function in the body - essentially how well our cells are functioning. This is important. 20-30% of our total Calories are burned via physical activity and 10-20% is expended through the energy cost or *thermic effect* of eating, known as *thermogenesis*.[85] It's generally agreed that to lose weight we have to create a gap between energy intake (what we eat), and energy expenditure: the sum total of these three contributions.

What most people typically do to create that gap is to burn more Calories through aerobic exercise while at the same time going on a diet – eating less food. This usually helps to create a *Calorie deficit*, and they lose weight. Great. But… as we know all too well, this weight loss tends to be both modest and short-lived – if it occurs at all. In fact, a study involving obese women showed that an exercise programme comprising of five, 45-minute sessions at 78% of their maximum heart-rate, for 12 weeks (more or less what we see most folks doing in the gym), had "no discernable effects on body composition"[86] – they didn't lose weight! Simply put, aerobic exercise is not a particularly effective weight loss tool – especially in women[87] (who, ironically, tend to gravitate to it most!).

The reason results are limited with this type of training is due in part to our metabolism. As we eat less food: (in many cases we are not even giving our body enough nourishment for normal function) the body retaliates by reducing our metabolism. This adaptation is an accepted part of weight loss[88,89,90]. Our bodies prefer balance, so if we reduce our energy intake, it will do it's best to expend less. So although we're being active, our body is gradually expending fewer Calories at rest. Why? Well, as far as our body is concerned, survival comes first, and if we're going through a famine (i.e. eating insufficient Calories), it's imperative that we preserve energy. As a result, cellular function slows down. We might experience a loss in body temperature, a drop in physical and mental energy, and low sex drive, amongst other things, as our body saves its energy for the essential tasks of keeping us alive. So we might be running every day on that treadmill, but with a reduced metabolism, we're fighting a losing battle. Like the example of Jill above, we've got to do more and more exercise just to break even.

WEIGHT LOSS VS. FAT LOSS
The other problem is that instead of burning our stored body fat for energy, our body will burn our muscle to make up the Calorie deficit[91,92]. Although we talk of weight loss, and get hung up on the number on the scales, the goal really is *fat loss*. We want to fill the gap between Calories burned and Calories eaten by burning our stored body fat so that we become leaner – or more 'toned' as people like to say.

Our body doesn't know that. Fat has more Calories per gram than does muscle so, from a survival point of view, it makes sense that our body should hang on to its fat stores to get us through the famine. Unless there is a demand to keep the muscle tissue, it burns our muscle instead. We see this muscle loss in marathon runners. Of course marathon runners lose fat as well, but since most people don't have the energy expenditure of a marathon runner, they burn muscle but never get to the fat stores. The result is that they find themselves 'skinny fat' despite doing lots of exercise. Not only are they *not* burning fat, they are losing muscle. Since muscle tissue is a contributor to our overall metabolic rate[93], this muscle loss results in a further drop in our metabolism. Remember, our metabolism accounts for 60-70% of our total Calories burned in a day, so a drop in metabolism is bad news for not only our health, but our fat-loss goals as well: as we're now expending much fewer Calories at rest.

> *"It appears that the combination of a large quantity of aerobic exercise with a very low calorie diet resulting in substantial loss of bodyweight may actually accelerate the decline in resting metabolic rate."*
>
> *(Poehlman et al, 1991)*[94]

When we finally can't take any more of the starvation diet (or lack of energy, or other symptoms of a sluggish metabolism) and begin to eat normally again (or even overeat as is usually seen after severe restriction[95]) guess what happens? Due to our lowered metabolism, our intake now exceeds our expenditure, we're now in a *Calorie surplus*, and we gain weight. We tried so hard! Running numerous times a week, spin classes, the lot. We were being "good" with the diet: no chocolate, no 'treats', fighting hunger ...and we *gained* weight. Sound familiar? It's heart-breaking, and so many folks are doing it. Don't get me wrong, you might lose weight for a while but if you are losing muscle and slowing your metabolism, there won't be a happy ending (and even with the short-term weight loss, it probably won't be a happy journey either).

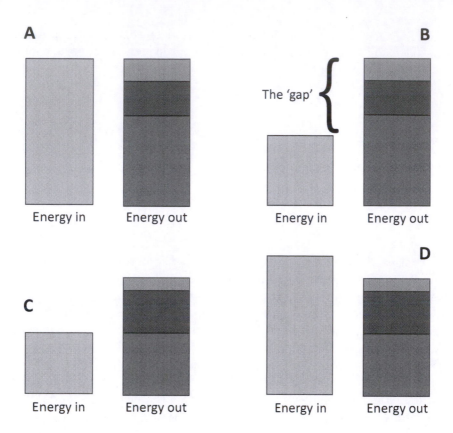

Yo-yo weight loss and weight gain.

A: Energy balance.

B: Calorie deficit but the gap is too big. The body receives insufficient nourishment and has no stimulus to hold on to its muscle mass.

C: The result is a drop in metabolism despite increased aerobic exercise. Weight loss may occur at this stage but muscle loss is also likely.

D: With a reduced metabolism, a return to normal eating results in a Calorie surplus and weight gain.

> *"Dieting is just depriving the body of energy. Obviously that works to an extent – but 'ramping up the system demands' is the more effective way to go."*
> *(Alwyn Cosgrove, fitness coach, author & gym owner)*

Metabolism is everything. Hopefully that's clear. Optimal metabolic function is essential for good energy and health. Moreover, if we keep our metabolism high, we burn more Calories *all the time* – even at rest. This allows us to create a subtle Calorie deficit while still consuming enough food to nourish the body. It's also crucial that we grow muscle (or at least preserve what we've got)[96]. Not only is our lean muscle mass a contributor to our overall metabolism, but by creating a demand for new muscle tissue, we're effectively telling our body not to burn the stuff for fuel – so we're more likely to burn fat instead.

Therefore, the goal of effective fat-loss training should be to increase our resting metabolism while building or preserving muscle tissue. When combined with an appropriate diet, this allows us to create a subtle gap between energy intake and energy expenditure that must be filled with fat.

How do we do that then?

1. Correct Nutrition

It bears repeating that you cannot out-train a bad diet – not for long anyway. Trying to burn fat without considering what we eat is unlikely to produce great results[97]. Similarly, while diet alone can work, best results are achieved when good nutrition is combined with an effective exercise programme[98].

I discussed nutrition in Part Two. Mindfully eat real food, and listen to the body's signals. Remember: hunger is not the enemy, and starvation is not the solution! If it helps, you can track Calories and macronutrients. *If* it helps!

While on the topic of exercise and metabolism it's important to recognise the importance of protein[99]. If we prioritise protein we do three things. First, protein is the most satiating nutrient, meaning we are less likely to overeat[100,101,102]. Second, protein has the greatest effect on the green *thermogenesis* section of our pie chart meaning we can increase that aspect of our energy expenditure[103]. Finally, protein, when combined with an appropriate exercise plan, helps to build and maintain muscle mass[104,105].

How much protein?
A protein intake greater than 1.05g per kilogram of your bodyweight each day is associated with greater muscle mass retention compared with diets with lower protein intakes[106], so for those tracking their nutrition, consider that your absolute minimum. While there still exist some myths about high protein intakes causing kidney damage, the research does not support this idea. In those with normal kidney function, higher protein intakes are considered safe[107]. Indeed, higher intakes (1.2g/kg) may be necessary to preserve metabolism[108], and are beneficial to body composition[109]. If you are participating in strength training (and for fat loss you should be!) it's likely that your protein requirements will be higher still with 1.8-2.0g/kg having been suggested[110,111]. Overall, a protein intake towards 2.0g per kg of bodyweight per day is appropriate. However, if you're highly trained and already have a somewhat lower body fat percentage, it has been suggested that a protein intake of 2.3-3.1g/kg of fat-free mass (bodyweight minus your body fat percentage) may be necessary depending on the severity of your caloric restriction[112]. If tracking nutrition isn't for you, these requirements can be met by eating a palm-sized source of protein at each meal.

2. Progressive strength training
After nutrition, your next most important tool when it comes to fat loss is strength training (also known as resistance training). While any sort of exercise will burn Calories, strength training increases (or at least preserves) our muscle tissue and helps us keep our metabolism up – benefits that we don't see with aerobic training alone[113,114,115]. In fact, in one study which compared diet only, diet plus aerobic exercise, and diet plus aerobics plus strength training, the addition of an aerobic training programme (30-50 minutes, three times a week for 12 weeks) didn't result in any more fat loss than just diet alone! The group that included strength training, however, lost 44% more fat than the diet-only group[116].

Strength training is incredibly diverse and can range from lifting just our own bodyweight, to using resistance bands, training with dumbbells and barbells as well as things like kettlebells and sandbags – basically anything heavy! Of particular use is short, high-intensity resistance training (think circuit training with only short recovery periods between exercises). This type of training may elevate our resting metabolism to a greater extent than does traditional strength training – even in a session lasting less than 15 minutes[117]. This is likely because, as well as creating that demand for muscle, training in this way allows us to benefit from an 'after-burn' effect known as *EPOC* (excess post-exercise oxygen consumption). This afterburn has the potential to elevate our metabolism for up to 38 hours afterwards[118] meaning we continue to burn extra

Calories long after we've stopped exercising. The magnitude of the afterburn effect depends primarily on the intensity of the training session[119,120,121]. So for ladies too, this means the resistance exercise must be challenging![122] No more 'triceps kickbacks' with 2kg dumbbells!

The 'toning' myth

On that note, while many people attempt to 'tone' specific body parts by exercising a specific muscle group (e.g. crunches to burn fat on the stomach, or triceps extensions for the 'bingo wings'), the research suggests that it's not possible to 'spot reduce' body fat[123,124,125]. We cannot choose parts of our body from which to lose fat; we can only burn fat in general. Our tendency to hang on to body fat in some places more than others is dictated in part by our genetics[126,127,128]. That being the case, it's more effective to focus on movements, not muscles. The fundamental movement patterns (squatting, lunging, bending, pushing, pulling) use large muscle groups: not only do they burn more Calories than a crunch or triceps kickback, but we also get stronger, more efficient movement for everyday life. If fat loss is your goal, stop wasting your time with crunches!

By performing exercises in *supersets* (performing two or more exercises then resting, rather than taking a rest period after every exercise) we can increase our energy expenditure both during and after the session while also saving ourselves some time[129]. Performing exercises explosively (i.e. fast and powerfully) may also help increase energy expenditure during and after sessions[130].

Strength training sessions can be anything from 15-45 minutes and are ideally performed 2-4 times per week. Frequency is important. When it comes to strength, even if we simply spread the same volume of training over three days rather than do it all in one session, we'll likely get better results[131].

Overall, the key point is this: if fat-loss is your goal, and you only have a few hours a week to train, you should only do traditional strength training or circuit-type training. Remember the importance of progressive overload: as we adapt and grow stronger, we must keep finding ways to increase the challenge – hence *progressive* strength training. Don't be that person who does the exact same workout every session for months on end! If it doesn't challenge you, it doesn't change you!

3. High-intensity interval training

If you happen to have some more time (and energy now that you're nourishing your body appropriately!) you could include some high-intensity interval training (often referred to as *HIIT*). This type of training involves exercising very hard for a very short period of time before recovering and repeating, and has been found to help with fat burning[132,133,134,135,136].

HIIT can be as simple as going outside and running a few short sprints interspersed with a walk back to the start line. We can use conventional gym machines like a treadmill, bike, or rowing machine, but anything goes: jumping rope, bodyweight exercises and boxing all offer great options. The key lies in getting the intensity right. HIIT does not mean alternating between a jog and a run every minute for 30 minutes. We have to work *hard*! To do this, we must keep the length of each interval, and the total duration of the interval workout, relatively short. Anything from 20-120 seconds is good for a work phase, with rest periods dependent on each individual.

Although we're unlikely to build much muscle with this type of training, we're still burning Calories, and the intensity means we can benefit from some serious metabolism-boosting afterburn.

4. Aerobic training
As we've seen, aerobic exercise tends not to be effective when it comes to fat-loss. It won't help us to build or preserve muscle mass nor will it boost our metabolic rate[137]. Besides, after adding 1-3 brief, high-intensity interval-training workouts to our strength-training programme, most of us probably won't have much time left in our week for more exercise.

Aerobic exercise does burn Calories though. So, if on top of our strength and interval training programmes, we still have time and energy for more exercise, now would be the time for some low or moderate intensity aerobic exercise – what people generally refer to as 'cardio'. These types of activities include any low-level physical activity up to around 70% of our maximum effort and can be a form of 'active recovery' for some.

Hopefully you can see the mistake most people make. Most people go straight for the cardio – low or high intensity. They end up burning Calories in the moment, but they don't maintain muscle and their metabolism suffers. When they get accustomed to it, they end up doing more and more and more until something breaks down (their body, their diet, their will). Their training is ineffective and their efforts go to waste. Ironically, despite sometimes being stuck in this cycle for years without fruition, many people are resistant to change when it comes to their training style. Many females in particular, still avoid strength training for fear of becoming too muscular. This is an unfortunate result of cultural and societal conditioning: it's both out-dated and unscientific.

"A concern for muscle as it pertains to exercise is one of the most important factors in changing body composition (body fat to lean tissue ratio). In other words, exercise designed to grow muscle (or at the very least, maintain it) – resistance exercise – is one of the most important factors in a program of exercise designed to change a person's ratio of body fat to total body weight."

(Alwyn Cosgrove, fitness coach, author & gym owner).

SUMMARY

In summary, an effective fat-loss training programme should prioritise:

1. Good nutrition
* Create a subtle Calorie deficit while providing enough Calories to support metabolism.
* Consume adequate protein to help satiety, boost thermogenesis and support muscle mass.

2. High-intensity strength training or traditional strength training
* Create a stimulus for the body to retain and grow muscle tissue.
* Support or boost metabolic rate.
* Promote fat-burning.
* Burn Calories.

3. High-intensity interval training
* Support or boost metabolic rate.
* Promote fat-burning.
* Burn Calories.

4. Aerobic exercise
* Burn some more Calories.

As for the exercises themselves, there are no magic ones. Find a programme that has a balance of fundamental movements. One more time, that means squatting, lunging, bending, pushing and pulling. While I cannot offer individualised exercise prescription in a book, you don't need to do it alone: find a coach you can trust and ask for help.

EXERCISING THE MIND

*"The single best investment we will ever make is investing
in our learning and self-development."*
(Robin Sharma, leadership expert and author)

The final piece I'd like to touch upon is exercise of a different type: exercising the mind. Exercising the mind (learning and being creative) can have a dramatic influence on the quality of our lives.

Unfortunately many people seem to be turned off by the idea of learning new things. Many people just do the minimum: they attain the credentials they need to get a job and leave it at that. Perhaps poor experiences with traditional learning methods at school are to blame. Perhaps it just seems like hard work or perhaps they don't believe they're capable of learning new things. Whatever the reason, it seems that many of us rarely bother to learn anything outwith what's expected for our job.

In her superb book, *Mindset*, Carol Dweck explains that when it comes to our capabilities, we tend to adopt one of two mindsets: a *fixed* mindset, or a *growth* mindset. Those who believe in the fixed mindset see traits as innate, inborn and fixed. Capability at a particular skill or task is something you either have or you don't. As a result, someone with a fixed mindset is reluctant to take on new challenges, preferring instead to stick to more familiar tasks. Since they see their capabilities as fixed, their traits represent who they are. Therefore, their self-esteem relies on their traits. Failure is seen as a disaster so when things go wrong it's everyone's fault but their own. As a personal trainer, I frequently see examples of a fixed mindset in the gym. These clients are wary of new exercises, they're afraid of mistakes so I have to tread carefully knowing that their self-esteem will be crushed if they try and fail at something new. They tend to talk about themselves in absolutes (e.g. "I have no coordination") or they decide that they are no good at a particular movement or exercise despite having only attempted one or two reps. That's when I often share one of my favourite quotes:

"You don't have to be great to start, but you have to start to be great."
(Zig Ziglar, author and motivational speaker)

This quote reflects the growth mindset. With the growth mindset, the person understands that important qualities can be cultivated: we *can* improve. Consequently when failure is encountered, it serves as an opportunity to learn and make progress. The person who adopts a growth mindset will tend to seek out increasingly difficult challenges, improving and growing each time. This person's self-esteem does not rely on their traits because their ability at any point in time is not *who* they are: they know they can get better and they tend to take responsibility for their own improvement. In the gym, clients with a growth mindset appreciate cues and coaching. They actively seek out feedback knowing that it is a tool for improvement.

> *"Every lapse doesn't spell doom. It's like anything else in the growth mindset – it's a reminder that you're an unfinished human being and a clue to how to do it better next time."*
>
> (Carol Dweck, author, Mindset)

The point is that no matter where we're at now (and regardless of our perceived intelligence) if we believe in the growth mindset, we can come to realise that we can learn and improve at anything …provided we're willing to invest the time. It's a fallacy that 'expert' performers in a given field are merely 'gifted' or 'talented'. In fact, with the exception of height, "individuals acquire virtually all of the distinguishing characteristics of expert performance through relevant activities (deliberate practice)"[138]. That doesn't mean we can all just decide to play tennis like Andy Murray and win Wimbledon next year. Clearly it takes a lot of work. It has been shown that true, elite level performance takes around 10000 hours or 10 years of deliberate practice to attain[139] and, as Malcolm Gladwell discusses in *Outliers*, while success might not be down to innate talent, sometimes we need to be in the right place at the right time. For example, as well as all his hard work and sacrifice, Andy Murray was introduced to tennis at a very young age and had the benefit of his mother being a tennis coach. So although it might not be time to rekindle that dream of winning Wimbledon, I'll say it again: we *can* improve. The plasticity of our brain means that it can be moulded and developed through deliberate practice – even in old age[140]. As Daniel Coyle explains in *The Talent Code*,

"(1) Every human movement, thought, or feeling is a precisely timed electric signal traveling through a chain of neurons—a circuit of nerve fibers.
(2) Myelin is the insulation that wraps these nerve fibers and increases signal strength, speed, and accuracy.
(3) The more we fire a particular circuit, the more myelin optimizes that circuit, and the stronger, faster, and more fluent our movements and thoughts become."

With deliberate practice we myelinate (insulate) the relevant circuits in our brain. The more myelin on a certain circuit, the more effective that circuit is at firing. So whether it's a circuit for driving a car, playing a musical instrument, reading, learning a language, doing mathematics or just using helpful thoughts (like silencing The Chimp!) – your mind is like your muscles: you can help it grow by using it in the right way.

I guess the question is: why bother putting in the effort to learn something new when we are comfortable as we are? Wouldn't it be easier to just sit and enjoy some TV?

WHY EXERCISE THE MIND?

One argument is the 'use it or lose it' theory. By 2050 it is estimated that the prevalence of Alzheimer's disease will quadruple from the 2006 worldwide prevalence of 26.6 million[141]. Studies have shown however, that cognitive decline is neither inevitable with ageing, nor irreversible[142]. Even in those already experiencing cognitive decline, marked improvements in things like memory can be achieved through training[143,144]. A relative of mine has Alzheimer's. Quality of life goes down fast. I do recognise though, that for most, learning new stuff *now* to avoid Alzheimer's disease in the *future* is hardly an inspiring proposition. So how about using your brain to feel happier today?

Work by the previously mentioned Mihaly Csikszentmihalyi (*Flow: The classic work on how to achieve happiness*), has shown that we're happiest when we're engaged in a 'flow' activity. Csikszentmihalyi's description of a flow activity sounds a lot like the state of 'deep' or deliberate practice required for learning. It requires our focus and attention. It's absorbing so our self-consciousness and worry about failure disappears. Our sense of time becomes distorted and, as I described when discussing mastery in Part One, the activity becomes it's own reward – we feel happy. Indeed, creativity and happiness are self-reinforcing[145]. Creativity is said to play an important role in our sense of wellbeing and is thought to be <u>as important as diet</u> for successful ageing[146]. The irony is that although we feel happiest when engaged in a flow activity like work or learning, most of us look forward to our passive leisure time.

> *"On the job people feel skilful and challenged, and therefore feel more happy, strong, creative, and satisfied. In their free time people feel that there is generally not much to do and their skills are not being used, and therefore they tend to feel more sad, weak, dull, and dissatisfied. Yet they would like to work less and spend more time in leisure."*
>
> *(Mihaly Csikszentmihalyi, Flow: The classic work on how to achieve happiness)*

It's like most things: what we *think* makes us happy (those pleasant experiences in the moment) rarely offers real fulfilment over time. A 'slob day' of watching movies with a takeaway dinner might be appealing from time to time but according to Csikszentmihalyi, we are happiest when we are engaged – when our "body or mind is stretched to its limits in a voluntary effort to accomplish something difficult and worthwhile."

GROWING OR DYING?

> *"When you stop growing you start dying."*
> *(William S. Burroughs, novelist)*

It's often said that everything in nature is either growing or dying, and although most of us are resigned to deteriorating with age (becoming fatter, sicker, and more tired) learning offers a powerful opportunity to grow. Learning means we can improve with age. We can develop new skills and abilities, not only becoming happier in the process, but also becoming a bigger, better version of ourselves.

If you are unhappy in your job, go learn a new skill and give yourself more options. It's remarkable how much we can actually learn for free nowadays! I'm no expert but I taught myself some basic Spanish by listening to free podcasts and I've learned to strum a few tunes on the guitar predominantly by watching and mimicking videos on

YouTube...over and over again. Not only were these fun experiences, they've made my life richer: the basic Spanish in particular proved very helpful during my backpacking adventure in Latin America. Make no mistake: neither one of these were easy – both were awkward and uncomfortable in the beginning (in fact, an initial attempt at learning the guitar seemed so difficult that I shelved the project for nearly three years!) By practising reading, I've been able to improve my speed and retention. By investing in books and listening to free podcasts, I've been able to absorb a vast amount of information on health and personal development – to the point where I felt capable of starting a blog, speaking in public and writing this book.

It has never been easier to get our hands on the best information and strategies in any field and to learn in a style that suits our own. You can learn anything you want: parenting, business, relationships, cooking, financial skills, sports, art, photography – anything! Not only will you be happier and keep your brain healthy, but you'll grow as a person and open yourself to new opportunities and new experiences. You might just find something you're truly passionate about!

"Too much undisciplined leisure time in which a person continually takes the course of least resistance gradually wastes a life. It ensures that a person's capacities stay dormant, that talents remain undeveloped, that the mind and spirit become lethargic and the heart is unfulfilled."
(Stephen Covey, educator & author, The 7 Habits of Highly Successful People)

The other option is to sit on the couch edging your way ever closer to the depressing dysfunction we assume is normal ageing. Unfortunately – and as with most things – those who need it the most do it the least, and those who need it the least do it the most. We see this with exercise and saving money and silencing The Chimp: those who need it the most do it the least; those who need it the least do it the most. So the smart get smarter, the wealthy get wealthier and the fit get fitter. A lot of people are left reciting their story. "I'm getting old", they say, "...I'm sure it's just my age." Which camp are you in? Are you growing or dying?

You *have* a choice. There are so many possibilities in life. There are so many people living fulfilled lives despite their challenging circumstances. You *can* learn, you *can* improve and you *can* grow.

PART THREE SUMMARY

* Movement is life: we must move well and we must move often.
* Pain and movement limitations are not merely a consequence of ageing and should be addressed.
* Focusing on performance enables us to find motivation through the concept of mastery.
* A performance goal can give us a sense of purpose in our training instead of just exercising to burn Calories.
* Exercise can be fun and doesn't need to be a beatdown.
* Working hard or long doesn't mean we're working effectively.
* Metabolism plays an important role in weight loss and fat loss.
* Aerobic exercise alone is not an effective fat loss tool.
* We cannot out-train a bad diet.
* Effective fat loss exercise prioritises progressive strength training.
* We cannot choose specific areas of our body from which to burn fat.
* High intensity interval training can assist fat-loss.
* Learning allows us to grow and become better with age.
* With practice we can learn and improve at almost anything.
* Using our brain can help prevent and reverse age-related cognitive decline.
* We are happiest when we are engaged in a 'flow' activity.
* Creativity and happiness are self-reinforcing.
* We can change our lives by learning something new.
* It has never been easier to find the best information and strategies in any field – and in a learning style that suits us.
* With most things, those who need it the most do it the least, and those who need it the least do it the most.

STEPPING FOREWARD

*"The amateur will be ready tomorrow. The sure sign of an amateur
is that he has a million plans and they all start tomorrow."*
(Steven Pressfield, Turning Pro)

WHAT HAPPENS NEXT?

If we want to make a change in our lives, ultimately we have to do something differently. We have to take action. It's too easy to read and learn something new, to nod along in agreement, and then go back to the same old habits and routine that didn't serve us well before.

We tell ourselves that the timing isn't ideal, that "life gets in the way" and that we'll start tomorrow or next month or next year. Inevitably we never get round to it. Time hurtles on. 'Ageing' takes over.
We repeat our story so much we eventually believe it to be true. "I was gonna, but..."
Then we get to the end.

*"Only at the moment of death do they recognize the fact that they have not lived.
Life has simply passed as if a dream, and death has come. Now there is no more time
to live – death is knocking on the door. And when there was time to live, you were
doing a thousand and one foolish things, wasting your time rather than living it."*

(Osho, spiritual teacher)

To be clear, I'm not suggesting we need all be Type A personality, driven goal-getters. Although I've been a bit like that myself at times, backpacking in Latin America taught me to relax more, to be more present and appreciative in the moment, and doing so has improved the quality of my life. I'm still ambitious but I feel happier. I'm also not suggesting that we need all aspire to some massive dream, aiming to change the world for millions – or make millions. We can change *our* world though. We can have stronger, happier energy on a day-to-day basis. We can enjoy a better quality of life and have a positive impact on those around us – be it our children, parents, work-colleagues, friends, or just the everyday people we share our world with. Energy is everything. To help you step forward, here is a summary of some of the main principles I've shared. Below, I've outlined a simple framework for action.

GET YOUR MIND RIGHT

Consider that you can choose how you respond to the circumstances and events in your life – nothing is *all* bad and challenges are both inevitable and necessary.

Recognise that rather than big one-off events, it tends to be the tiny things you do regularly – your habits – that dictate the quality of your life.

You can enhance your motivation through autonomy, mastery and a deep sense of purpose – your 'why'.

NOURISH YOUR BODY

Base your diet on real, whole food that can be prepared at home.

Eat an appropriate amount by practicing mindful eating and avoiding unnecessary food restriction.

Respect the impact sleep, time in nature, and social community have on your overall energy and wellbeing.

MOVE!

Move your body. Move well and move often. Pick a performance goal and have some fun with your movement. Consider the effectiveness of your exercise – especially with regards to fat-loss.

Move your mind. Use your brain. Explore some creative pursuits and learn something new. Adopt a growth mindset and stretch your capabilities.

WHAT TO DO NOW

Step 1: Consider your 'why'
You want to improve your energy, your life, your happiness. Like most people, you've probably tried before. While the process might be simple, it won't necessarily be easy. There will be challenges. As we've seen, having an inspiring purpose – a 'why' – is critical. Reasons precede results.

Try connecting your goal to what you value most in life. Find an emotional reason that keeps you fired up. Write it down and look at it daily. Discipline is remembering what you want.

Step 2: Identify your limiting factor
Which of your thoughts, habits and behaviours are holding you back from your goal? Of these, which is your *biggest limiting factor*?

People get hung up on minutiae like the optimal time of day to exercise, which so-called 'superfoods' they should be consuming, or the timing of their food intake. Yet none of these are likely to be your biggest limiting factor. More likely you are simply not eating an appropriate amount of food, or your exercise programme is ineffective or inconsistent. Perhaps your sleep quality is poor. Maybe you surround yourself with people who tear you down more than they lift you up. Have a look in the mirror – maybe you do it to yourself. Maybe you need to tidy up your environment – nutritionally, socially, physically – what are you surrounding yourself with? Do shopping or leisure time habits need a little tweaking? Do you need a better system that allows you to eat and move well?

Whatever it is, find your biggest limiting factor and take ownership of it. When you take responsibility for it, you give yourself the power to change it. We often complain that we just don't have the time. Aside from being outwith our control, I'm not convinced that time is our biggest limiting factor. The reality is we spend our time, money and energy on what we value most.

Step 3: Choose one action step or new habit

Pick one, easy behaviour you can implement that will begin to address your biggest limiting factor. Follow the guidelines outlined in the habits section of Part One (choose one easy, measureable habit-change and check in daily).

For instance, if you are full of negative self-talk, you might want to start by noticing and tallying those instances of Chimp Chatter. If your limiting factor is overeating, you might start by placing your focus on eating more slowly and mindfully. If you have movement issues, you could focus on performing one mobility exercise every day. If you want to learn something new, you could start the habit of studying for five minutes every evening.

Step 4: Practice

The goal is *progression* not perfection. Remember, we *can* improve. Everything is a practice. Practice your habit. If you slip up, practice self-compassion! Review your 'why', wipe the slate clean, and get back on track immediately. Whether or not our habits are helpful, like it or not, we're always reinforcing *something*. If you never really move your body or utilise the range of motion in your joints, by default you're just practising and reinforcing those few positions that you do use. Inevitably, through this practice, you'll become really good at your poor posture and having tight muscles and stiff joints!

If we are always practising something, it would be wise to practice habits that serve us.

Step 5: Repeat

When the new behaviour becomes habitual, identify your next biggest limiting factor, set an appropriate behaviour goal, and practice that too. In this way, step-by-step, inch-by-inch we build our energy and enhance the quality of our life.

Really there is no other way. The alternative, the path of least resistance, rarely leads us anywhere worthwhile. The 'easy life' is a myth: more likely all we get is complacency, apathy and eventually regret. Expending effort, struggling, failing, and eventually overcoming obstacles on a path towards something valuable to us, is where we find the greatest rewards. Appreciate the journey. You're in it for the long haul.

> *"If you're willing to do only what's easy, life will be hard.*
> *But if you're willing to do what's hard, life will be easy."*
> *(T. Harv Eker, author, businessman and motivational speaker)*

YOU CAN

I guess if I could leave you with one final message, it's that *you* can. Regardless of what has happened before, regardless of your circumstances, you can. Recognise that you're *already* a worthy person. You are *already* enough. Recognise if you want to grow or change or improve, you can.

You *can* choose responsibility over victimhood.
You *can* choose to let go of your story.
You *can* choose to make a change.
You *can* choose to think in more helpful ways.
You *can* grow and improve. At anything.
You *can* form new habits.
You *can* become fit and healthy.
You *can* lose fat.
You *can* become stronger.
You *can* learn new skills.
You *can* develop your virtues – courage, compassion, patience, persistence.
You *can* step outside your comfort zone.
You *can* make a difference.
You *can* be happy.
You *can* become the best version of yourself.

Start now.
The time will pass anyway.

"In order for us to become truly happy,
that which we can become, we must become."

(Abraham Maslow, psychologist)

Energy is everything.

Always Keep Reaching!

Want more? Visit www.MikeMacDonald.co.uk/EiE to sign up to my email list and receive bonus goodies!

BIBLIOGRAPHY

Part One

Man's Search for Meaning – Viktor Frankl
Meditations – Marcus Aurelius
Finding Joe (movie) – Patrick Takaya Solomon
What Happy People Know – Dr Dan Baker & Cameron Stauth
Flow: The classic work on how to achieve happiness – Mihaly Csikszentmihalyi
The Power of Habit – Charles Duhigg
The Power of Less – Leo Babauta
The Compound Effect – Darren Hardy
Drive: The surprising truth about what motivates us – Daniel Pink
The 7 Habits of Highly Effective People – Steven Covey
The Secret to Success – Eric Thomas
The Total Money Makeover Workbook – Dave Ramsey

Part Two

Diet Recovery 2 – Matt Stone
Deep Nutrition – Catherine & Luke Shanahan
The Dark Side of Fat Loss – Sean Croxton
In Defence of Food – Michael Pollan
WholeHealthSource.blogspot.co.uk – Stephan Guyenet
The End of Overeating – David Kessler
The Harcombe Diet – Zoe Harcombe
Influence: The psychology of persuasion – Robert Cialdini
The Way of The Peaceful Warrior – Dan Millman
The War of Art – Steven Pressfield
Turning Pro – Steven Pressfield
Yes: 50 Secrets from the science of persuasion – Goldstein, Martin & Cialdini
Mindless Eating – Brian Wansink
The Kick-Ass Life Podcast – David Wood

Part Three

Becoming a Supple Leopard: The ultimate guide to resolving pain, preventing injury, and optimizing athletic performance – Dr Kelly Starett
Athletic Body in Balance – Gray Cook
Movement – Gray Cook
The Results Fitness Ultimate Fat Loss Programming and Coaching System – Alwyn & Rachel Cosgrove
Mindset – Carol Dweck
Outliers: The story of success – Malcolm Gladwell
The Talent Code – Daniel Coyle

Stepping Forward

Courage: The joy of living dangerously – Osho

1   Wiseman, R. University of Bristol http://www.quirkology.com/UK/Experiment_resolution.shtml
2   Lally et al. 2010. How are habits formed: Modelling habit formation in the real world. European Journal of Social Psychology 40(6): 998–1009
3   WHO 2003: http://www.who.int/chp/knowledge/publications/adherence_full_report.pdf
4   As reported by CBC News Canada: http://www.cbc.ca/news/canada/story/2006/02/10/polarbear-mom060210.html
5   From ABC News: http://abcnews.go.com/US/superhero-woman-lifts-car-off-dad/story?id=16907591#.UMay9Hfeba4
6   Ravnskov, U. 2002. A hypothesis out-of-date: The diet–heart idea Journal of Clinical Epidemiology 55:1057–1063
7   Krumholz et al. 1994. Lack of Association Between Cholesterol and Coronary Heart Disease Mortality and Morbidity and All-Cause Mortality in Persons Older Than 70 Years. JAMA. 272(17): 1335-1340
8   Ravnskov, U. 1992. Cholesterol lowering trials in coronary heart disease: frequency of citation and outcome. BMJ 305(6844):15–19.
9   Schatz et al. 2001. Cholesterol and all-cause mortality in elderly people from the Honolulu Heart Program: a cohort study. The Lancet 358(9279):351-355
10 Okayama et al. 1993. Changes in Total Serum Cholesterol and Other Risk Factors for Cardiovascular Disease in Japan, 1980–1989. Int. J. Epidemiol 22(6):1038-1047
11 Ravnskov, U. 1998. The Questionable Role of Saturated and Polyunsaturated Fatty Acids in Cardiovascular Disease. J Clin Epidemiol 51(6):443–460
12 Simopoulos, AP. 2008. The Importance of the Omega-6/Omega-3 Fatty Acid Ratio in Cardiovascular Disease and Other Chronic Diseases. Exp Biol Med (Maywood) 233(6):674-688
13 Sørensen, LB. et al. 2003. Effect of sensory perception of foods on appetite and food intake: a review of studies on humans. Int J Obes Relat Metab Disord. 27(10):1152-66.
14 http://wholehealthsource.blogspot.co.uk/2012/03/food-reward-approaching-scientific.html
15 Alsiö et al. 2012. Feed-forward mechanisms: addiction-like behavioral and molecular adaptations in overeating. Front Neuroendocrinol. 33(2):127-39
16 Erdmann et al. 2008. Development of hyperinsulinemia and insulin resistance during the early stage of weight gain. Am J Physiol Endocrinol Metab. 294(3):E568-75
17 DeFronzo, RA. & Ferrannini, E. 1991. Insulin Resistance: A Multifaceted Syndrome Responsible for NIDDM, Obesity, Hypertension, Dyslipidemia, and Atherosclerotic Cardiovascular Disease. Diabetes Care 14(3):173-194
18 Myers MG, Cowley MA, Münzberg H. 2008. Mechanisms of leptin action and leptin resistance. Annu Rev Physiol. 70:537-56.
19 Morris, DL. & Rui, L. 2009. Recent advances in understanding leptin signaling and leptin resistance. American Journal of Physiology - Endocrinology and Metabolism 297:E1247-E1259
20 Tomiyama et al. 2010. Low Calorie Dieting Increases Cortisol. Psychosom Med. 72(4):357–364.
21 McLean JA, Barr SI, Prior JC. 2001. Cognitive dietary restraint is associated with higher urinary cortisol excretion in healthy premenopausal women. Am J Clin Nutr. 73(1):7-12.
22 Rideout CA, Linden W, Barr SI. 2006. High cognitive dietary restraint is associated with increased cortisol excretion in postmenopausal women. J.Gerontol A Biol Sci Med Sci. 61(6):628-33.
23 Gailliot et al. 2007. Self-control relies on glucose as a limited energy source: willpower is more than a metaphor. J Pers Soc Psychol. 92(2):325-36.
24 Gailliot, MT & Baumeister, RF. The physiology of willpower: linking blood glucose to self-control. Pers Soc Psychol Rev. 11(4):303-27
25 Kandiah et al. 2006. Stress influences appetite and comfort food preferences in college women. Nutrition Research 26(3):118–123
26 Epel et al. 2001. Stress may add bite to appetite in women: a laboratory study of stress-induced cortisol and eating behaviour. Psychoneuroendocrinology 26 (1):37–49
27 Wardle et al. 2000. Stress, dietary restraint and food intake. Journal of Psychosomatic Research 48(2):195–202
28 Stewart TM, Williamson DA, White MA. Rigid vs. flexible dieting: association with eating disorder symptoms in nonobese women. Appetite. 2002 Feb;38(1):39 44.
29 Meule et al. 2011. Food cravings mediate the relationship between rigid, but not flexible control of eating behavior and dieting success. Appetite. 57(3):582–584
30 Robinson et al. (2013) Eating attentively: a systematic review and meta-analysis of the effect of food intake memory and awareness on eating. American Society for Nutrition, April 2013
31 Karl JP, Young AJ, Montain SJ. 2011. Eating rate during a fixed-portion meal does not affect postprandial appetite and gut peptides or energy intake during a subsequent meal. Physiology & Behavior 102(5):524–531
32 Andrade AM, Greene GW, Melanson KJ; 2008. Eating Slowly Led to Decreases in Energy Intake within Meals in Healthy Women. Journal of the American Dietetic Association. 108(7):1186–1191
33 Hill SW & McCutcheon NB. 1984. Contributions of obesity, gender, hunger, food preference, and body size to bite size, bite speed, and rate of eating Appetite 5(2):73-83
34 Alsiö et al. 2012. Feed-forward mechanisms: addiction-like behavioral and molecular adaptations in overeating. Front Neuroendocrinol. Apr 33(2):127-39
35 Sørensen et al. 2003. Effect of sensory perception of foods on appetite and food intake: a review of studies on humans. Int J Obes Relat Metab Disord. Oct 27(10):1152-66.
36 Fuhrman et al. 2010. Changing perceptions of hunger on a high nutrient density diet. Nutrition Journal 9:51
37 Madden et al. 2012. Eating in response to hunger and satiety signals is related to BMI in a nationwide sample of 1601 mid-age New Zealand women. Public Health Nutrition. Mar 23:1-8
38 Herbert et al. 2013. Intuitive eating is associated with interoceptive sensitivity. Effects on body mass index. Appetite 70(1):22–30

39   Smith, T. & Hawks, SR. 2006. Intuitive eating, diet composition, and the meaning of food in healthy weight population. American Journal of Health Education 37(3):130-136

40   Denny et al. 2013. Intuitive eating in young adults. Who is doing it, and how is it related to disordered eating behaviors? Appetite. 2013 Jan;60(1):13-9.

41   Hawks et al. 2005. The relationship between intuitive eating and health indicators among college women. American Journal of Health Education 36(6):331-336

42   van't Riet et al. 2011. The importance of habits in eating behaviour. An overview and recommendations for future research. Appetite 57(3):585–596

43   Knutson et al. 2007. The metabolic consequences of sleep deprivation. Sleep Medicine Reviews (2007)11:163–178

44   Taheri et al. 2004. Short sleep duration is associated with reduced leptin, elevated ghrelin, and increased body mass index. PLoS Med 1(3): e62.

45   Van Cauter et al. 2007. Impact of Sleep and Sleep Loss on Neuroendocrine and Metabolic Function. Horm Res 2007;67(suppl 1):2–9

46   Spiegel et al. 2004. Leptin Levels Are Dependent on Sleep Duration: Relationships with Sympathovagal Balance, Carbohydrate Regulation, Cortisol, and Thyrotropin. J Clin Endocrinol Metab 89: 5762–5771, 2004

47   Brondel et al. 2010. Acute partial sleep deprivation increases food intake in healthy men. Am J Clin Nutr 2010;91:1550–9

48   Yaggi et al. 2006. Sleep Duration as a Risk Factor for the Development of Type 2 Diabetes. Diabetes Care 29:657–661, 2006

49   Gottlieb et al. 2005. Association of Sleep Time With Diabetes Mellitus and Impaired Glucose Tolerance. Arch Intern Med; 205; 165:863-868

50   Spiegel et al. 2009. Effects of poor and short sleep on glucose metabolism and obesity risk. Nat. Rev. Endocrinol. 5, 253–261 (2009)

51   Knutson & Van Cauter. 2008. Associations between Sleep Loss and Increased Risk of Obesity and Diabetes. Ann. N.Y. Acad. Sci. 1129: 287–304

52   Donga et al. 2010. A Single Night of Partial Sleep Deprivation Induces Insulin Resistance in Multiple Metabolic Pathways in Healthy Subjects. J Clin Endocrinol Metab 95: 2963–2968, 2010

53   Irwin et al. 2006. Sleep Deprivation and Activation of Morning Levels of Cellular and Genomic Markers of Inflammation 2006 30 subjects. Arch Intern Med 2006; 166:1756-1762

54   Meier-Ewert et al. 2004. Effect of Sleep Loss on C-Reactive Protein, an Inflammatory Marker of Cardiovascular Risk. Am Coll Cardiol 2004;43:678–83

55   Durmer, JS. & Dinges, DF. 2005. Neurocognitive Consequences of Sleep Deprivation. Semin Neurol. 25(1):117-129

56   Capellini et al. 2009. Does Sleep Play a Role in Memory Consolidation? A Comparative Test. PLoS ONE 4(2): e4609.

57   Lim & Dinges, 2008. Sleep Deprivation and Vigilant Attention. Ann. N.Y. Acad. Sci. 1129: 305–322 (2008)

58   Wojnar et al. 2009 Sleep problems and suicidality in the National Comorbidity Survey Replication. Journal of Psychiatric Research 43 (2009) 526–531

59   Berman MG, Jonides J, Kaplan S. 2008. The Cognitive Benefits of Interacting With Nature. Psychological Science 2008 vol. 19 (12):1207-1212

60   Korpela et al. 2010. Favorite green, waterside and urban environments, restorative experiences and perceived health in Finland. Health Promot. Int. (2010) 25 (2): 200-209.

61   Ulrich et al. 1991. Stress recovery during exposure to natural and urban environments. Journal of Environmental Psychology Volume 11 (3) September 1991:201–230

62   Berman et al. 2012. Interacting with nature improves cognition and affect for individuals with depression. Journal of Affective Disorders140(3): 300–305

63   Maller et al. 2006. Healthy nature healthy people: 'contact with nature' as an upstream health promotion intervention for populations. Health Promot. Int. (March 2006) 21(1): 45-54.

64   Maas et al. 2006. Green space, urbanity, and health: how strong is the relation? J Epidemiol Community Health 2006;60:587-592

65   Holick, M.F. 2011. Vitamin D deficiency in 2010: Health benefits of vitamin D and sunlight: a D-bate. Nature Reviews Endocrinology 7:73-75

66   Holick, M.F. 2008. Vitamin D and Sunlight: Strategies for Cancer Prevention and Other Health Benefits. CJASN September 2008 3(5): 1548-1554

67   Baumeister, RF & Leary, MR. 1995. The need to belong: Desire for interpersonal attachments as a fundamental human motivation. Psychological Bulletin, 117(3): 497-529.

68   Andrew MK, Mitnitski AB, Rockwood K. 2008. Social Vulnerability, Frailty and Mortality in Elderly People. PLoS ONE 3(5)

69   Holt-Lunstad J, Smith TB, Layton JB. 2010. Social Relationships and Mortality Risk: A Meta-analytic Review. PLoS Med 7(7)

70   Helliwell, JF. & Putnam, RD. 2004. The social context of well–being. Phil. Trans. R. Soc. Lond. 359(1449): 1435-1446

71   Kawachi I , Kennedy BP, Glass, R. 1999. Social capital and self-rated health: a contextual analysis. American Journal of Public Health August 1999: Vol. 89, No. 8, pp. 1187-1193.

72   Christakis & Fowler. 2007. The Spread of Obesity in a Large Social Network over 32 Years. N Engl J Med 357: 370-379

73   Ido Portal on Paleo Diet, CrossFit, Gymnastics, Motivation, Movement & More - RawBrahs. http://www.youtube.com/watch?v=aLogFAbTIDI [accessed online 12th June 2013]

74   Tabata et al. 1996. Effects of moderate-intensity endurance and high-intensity intermittent training on anaerobic capacity and VO2max. Medicine & Science in Sports & Exercise 28 (10): 1327-1330

75   Helgerud et al. 2007. Aerobic high-intensity intervals improve VO2max more than moderate training. Med Sci Sports Exerc. 2007 39(4): 665-71.

76   Man-Gyoon Lee et al. 2012. Effects of high-intensity exercise training on body composition, abdominal fat loss, and cardiorespiratory fitness in middle-aged Korean females. Applied Physiology, Nutrition, and Metabolism, 2012, 37(6): 1019-1027

77   Tremblay A, Simoneau J-A, Bouchard, C. 1994. Impact of exercise intensity on body fatness and skeletal muscle metabolism. Metabolism 43(7): 814–818

78   Yoshioka et al. 2001. Impact of high-intensity exercise on energy expenditure, lipid oxidation and body fatness. International Journal of Obesity and Related Metabolic Disorders : Journal of the International Association for the Study of Obesity 2001, 25(3): 332-339

79   Rognmo et al. 2004. High intensity aerobic interval exercise is superior to moderate intensity exercise for increasing aerobic capacity in patients with coronary artery disease. European Journal of Preventive Cardiology 11(3): 216-222

80   Wisløff et al. 2007. Superior Cardiovascular Effect of Aerobic Interval Training Versus Moderate Continuous Training in Heart Failure Patients A Randomized Study. Circulation 2007; 115: 3086-3094

81   van den Ende et al. 1996. Comparison of high and low intensity training in well controlled rheumatoid arthritis. Results of a randomised clinical trial. Ann Rheum Dis 1996 55: 798-805

82   Lee I-M, Hsieh C-C, Paffenbarger, RS. 1995. Exercise Intensity and Longevity in Men: The Harvard Alumni Health Study. JAMA. 1995;273(15):1179-1184

83   Laursen, PB & Jenkins, DG. 2002. The Scientific Basis for High-Intensity Interval Training. Sports Medicine 32(1): 53-73

84   From 'The Results Fitness Ultimate Fat Loss Programming and Coaching System' by Rachel & Alwyn Cosgrove with Craig Rasmussen & Mike Wunsch. Cosgrove FAST Systems, Inc. 2001. www.ResultsUniversity.com

85   Ravussin et al. 1986. Determinants of 24-hour energy expenditure in man. Methods and results using a respiratory chamber. J Clin Invest. 1986 December; 78(6): 1568–1578.

86   Utter et al. 1998. Influence of diet and/or exercise on body composition and cardiorespiratory fitness in obese women. Int J Sport Nutr. 1998 Sep;8(3):213-22.

87   Gleim GW. 1993. Exercise is not an effective weight loss modality in women. J Am Coll Nutr. 1993 12(4): 363-7.

88   Major et al. 2007. Clinical significance of adaptive thermogenesis. International Journal of Obesity 31: 204–212.

89   Doucet et al. 2001. Evidence for the existence of adaptive thermogenesis during weight loss. Br J Nutr. 85(6): 715-23.

90   Heilbronn et al. 2006. Effect of 6-Month Calorie Restriction on Biomarkers of Longevity, Metabolic Adaptation, and Oxidative Stress in Overweight Individuals A Randomized Controlled Trial. JAMA. 295(13): 1539-1548

91   Stiegler & Cunliffe. 2006. Sports Medicine. The Role of Diet and Exercise for the Maintenance of Fat-Free Mass and Resting Metabolic Rate During Weight Loss. 36(3): 239-262

92   Chaston et al. 2007. Changes in fat-free mass during significant weight loss: a systematic review. International Journal of Obesity 31:743–750

93   Illner et al. 2000. Metabolically active components of fat free mass and resting energy expenditure in nonobese adults. American Journal of Physiology - Endocrinology and Metabolism 278: E308-E315

94   Poehlman ET, Melby CL, Goran MI. 1991. The impact of exercise and diet restriction on daily energy expenditure. Sports Med. 1991 Feb;11(2):78-101.

95   Dulloo et al. 2012. How dieting makes some fatter: from a perspective of human body composition autoregulation. Proc Nutr Soc. 71(3): 379-89.

96   Wolfe, RR. 2006. The underappreciated role of muscle in health and disease. Am J Clin Nutr. 84(3): 475-482

97   Miller WC, Koceja DM, Hamilton EJ. 1997. A meta-analysis of the past 25 years of weight loss research using diet, exercise or diet plus exercise intervention. Int J Obes Relat Metab Disord. 1997 Oct;21(10):941-7.

98   Kraemer et al. 1999. Influence of exercise training on physiological and performance changes with weight loss in men. Med Sci Sports Exerc. 1999 Sep;31(9):1320-9.

99   Soenen et al. Relatively high-protein or 'low-carb' energy-restricted diets for body weight loss and body weight maintenance? Physiol Behav. 2012 Oct 10;107(3):374-80.

100 Halton et al. 2004. The Effects of High Protein Diets on Thermogenesis, Satiety and Weight Loss: A Critical Review. Journal of the American College of Nutrition 23(5)

101 Soenen & Westerterp-Plantenga. 2008. Proteins and satiety: implications for weight management. Curr Opin Clin Nutr Metab Care. 2008 Nov;11(6):747-51.

102 Johnstone, A. 2012. Safety and efficacy of high-protein diets for weight loss. *Proceedings of the Nutrition Society* 71(2): 339-349

103 Westerterp, KR. 2004. Diet induced thermogenesis. Nutrition & Metabolism 1(5)

104 Bosse, JD. & Dixon, BM. 2012. Dietary protein to maximize resistance training: a review and examination of protein spread and change theories. Journal of the International Society of Sports Nutrition 9(42)

105 Stiegler & Cunliffe. 2006. The Role of Diet and Exercise for the Maintenance of Fat-Free Mass and Resting Metabolic Rate During Weight Loss. Sports Medicine 36(3): 239-262

106 Krieger et al. 2006. Effects of variation in protein and carbohydrate intake on body mass and composition during energy restriction: a meta-regression 1. Am J Clin Nutr. 2006 Feb;83(2):260-74.

107 Manninen, A.H. 2004. High-Protein Weight Loss Diets and Purported Adverse Effects: Where is the Evidence? J Int Soc Sports Nutr. 2004; 1(1): 45–51.

108 Soenen et al. 2013. Normal protein intake is required for body weight loss and weight maintenance, and elevated protein intake for additional preservation of resting energy expenditure and fat free mass. J Nutr. 2013 May;143(5):591-6.

109 Westerterp-Plantenga et al. 2012. Dietary protein - its role in satiety, energetics, weight loss and health. Br J Nutr. 2012 Aug;108 Suppl 2:S105-12.

110 Tarnopolsky et al. 1992. Evaluation of protein requirements for trained strength athletes. J Appl Physiol. 1992 Nov;73(5):1986-95.

111 Phillips SM & Van Loon LJ. Dietary protein for athletes: from requirements to optimum adaptation. J Sports Sci. 2011;29 Suppl 1:S29-38.

112 Helms et al. 2013. A Systematic Review of Dietary Protein During Caloric Restriction in Resistance Trained Lean Athletes: A Case for Higher Intakes. Int J Sport Nutr Exerc Metab. 2013 Oct 2. [Epub ahead of print]

113 Ryan et al. 1995. Resistive training increases fat-free mass and maintains RMR despite weight loss in postmenopausal women. Journal of Applied Physiology September 1, 1995 79(3): 818-823

114 Bryner et al. 1999. Effects of resistance vs. aerobic training combined with an 800 calorie liquid diet on lean body mass and resting metabolic rate. Nutr. 1999 Apr;18(2):115-21.

115 Hunter et al. 2008. Resistance training conserves fat-free mass and resting energy expenditure following weight loss. Obesity (Silver Spring). 2008 May;16(5):1045-51.

116 Kramer et al. 1999. Influence of exercise training on physiological and performance changes with weight loss in men. Med. Sci. Sports Exerc., 31(9): 1320-1329

117 Paoli et al. 2012. High-Intensity Interval Resistance Training (HIRT) influences resting energy expenditure and respiratory ratio in non-dieting individuals. J Transl Med. 2012 Nov 24;10:237.

118 Schuenke et al. 2002. Effect of an acute period of resistance exercise on excess post-exercise oxygen consumption: implications for body mass management. Eur J Appl Physiol. 86(5): 411-7

119 Sedlock et al. 1989. Effect of exercise intensity and duration on postexercise energy expenditure. Med Sci Sports Exerc. 1989 Dec;21(6):662-6.

120 Phelain et al. 1997. Postexercise energy expenditure and substrate oxidation in young women resulting from exercise bouts of different intensity. J Am Coll Nutr. 1997 Apr;16(2):140-6.

121 Thornton, MK & Potteiger, JA. 2002. Effects of resistance exercise bouts of different intensities but equal work on EPOC. Med Sci Sports Exerc. 2002 Apr;34(4):715-22.

122 Osterberg KL & Melby CL. 2000. Effect of acute resistance exercise on postexercise oxygen consumption and resting metabolic rate in young women. Int J Sport Nutr Exerc Metab. 2000 Mar;10(1):71-81.

123 Vispute et al. 2011. The effect of abdominal exercise on abdominal fat. J Strength Cond Res. 25(9): 2559-64

124 Katch et al. 1984. Effects of Sit up Exercise Training on Adipose Cell Size and Adiposity. Research Quarterly for Exercise and Sport 55(3): 242-247

125 Ramirez-Campillo et al. 2013. Regional Fat Changes Induced by Localized Muscle Endurance Resistance Training. J Strength Cond Res. 27(8): 2219-2224.

126 Selby et al. 1990. Genetic and behavioral influences on body fat distribution. Int J Obes. 14(7): 593-602.

127   Malis et al. 2005. Total and regional fat distribution is strongly influenced by genetic factors in young and elderly twins. Obes Res. 13(12): 2139-45

128   Herrera et al. 2011. Genetics and epigenetics of obesity. Maturitas 69(1): 41–49

129   Kelleher et al. 2010. The metabolic costs of reciprocal supersets vs. traditional resistance exercise in young recreationally active adults. J Strength Cond Res. 2010 Apr;24(4):1043-51.

130   Mazzetti et al. 2007. Effect of explosive versus slow contractions and exercise intensity on energy expenditure. Med Sci Sports Exerc. 2007 Aug;39(8):1291-301.

131   McLester et al. 2000. Comparison of 1 Day and 3 Days Per Week of Equal-Volume Resistance Training in Experienced Subjects. The Journal of Strength and Conditioning Research 14(3).

132   Irving et al. 2008. Effect of exercise training intensity on abdominal visceral fat and body composition. Med Sci Sports Exerc. 2008 Nov;40(11):1863-72.

133   Bryner et al. 1997. The effects of exercise intensity on body composition, weight loss, and dietary composition in women. J Am Coll Nutr. 1997 Feb;16(1):68-73.

134   Tremblay et al. 1994. Impact of exercise intensity on body fatness and skeletal muscle metabolism. Metabolism. 1994 Jul;43(7):814-8.

135   Boutcher SH. 2011. High-intensity intermittent exercise and fat loss. J Obes. 2011.

136   Talanian et al. 2007. Two weeks of high-intensity aerobic interval training increases the capacity for fat oxidation during exercise in women. J Appl Physiol. 2007 Apr;102(4):1439-47.

137   Broeder et al. 1992. The effects of aerobic fitness on resting metabolic rate. Am J Clin Nutr. 1992 Apr;55(4):795-801.

138   Ericsson KA, Krampe RT, Tesch-Romer, C. 1993. The Role of Deliberate Practice in the Acquisition of Expert Performance. Psychological Review 1993, 100(3): 363-406

139   Ericsson KA, Krampe RT, Tesch-Romer, C. 1993. The Role of Deliberate Practice in the Acquisition of Expert Performance. Psychological Review 1993 100(3): 363-406

140   Anderson, S & Kraus, N. 2013. Auditory Training: Evidence for Neural Plasticity in Older Adults. Perspectives on Hearing and Hearing Disorders: Research and Diagnostics 17(1): 37-57

141   Brookmeyer et al. 2007. Forecasting the global burden of Alzheimer's disease. Alzheimer's & Dementia: The Journal of the Alzheimer's Association 3(3): 186-191

142   Thompson, G & Foth, D. 2005. Cognitive-Training Programs for Older Adults: What Are they and Can they Enhance Mental Fitness? Educational Gerontology 31(8): 603-626

143   Mahncke et al. 2006. Memory enhancement in healthy older adults using a brain plasticity-based training program: A randomized, controlled study. PNAS 103(33): 12523-12528

144   Ball, et al. 2002. Effects of Cognitive Training Interventions With Older Adults: A Randomized Controlled Trial. JAMA 288(18): 2271-2281

145   Pannells, TC & Claxton, AF. 2008. Happiness, Creative Ideation, and Locus of Control. Creativity Research Journal. 20(1): 67-71

146   Chan, J. 2005. The Necessity of Creativity. Paper presented at the Business/Higher Education Round Table Emerging Skills Summit 2020 and Beyond, 22 November 2005

Printed in Great Britain
by Amazon.co.uk, Ltd.,
Marston Gate.

TEACH YOURSELF

CROQUET

INCLUDING GAMES FOR THE GARDEN AND THE CROQUET ASSOCIATION RULES

Don Gaunt

Hodder & Stoughton

LONDON SYDNEY AUCKLAND

British Library Cataloguing in Publication Data

Gaunt, Don
  Teach yourself croquet.
  I. Title
  796.35

ISBN 0-340-56528-4

First published 1992

Typeset by Rowland Phototypesetting Ltd, Bury St Edmunds, Suffolk
Printed in Great Britain for the educational publishing division of Hodder & Stoughton Ltd, Mill Road, Dunton Green, Sevenoaks, Kent by Clays Ltd, St Ives plc, Bungay, Suffolk

———— CONTENTS ————

About the author

Don Gaunt first started playing croquet in the early 70s when he discovered a set in the basement at work. With some friends, he worked out the rules and started to play. Like many people, he had no idea that the game was played nationally and it wasn't until he moved to Ipswich in 1979 and joined the club there that he began to play seriously.

Since that time he has played in many events, both nationally and internationally. He was chairman of the Ipswich Croquet Club for several years before moving to Gloucestershire where he joined both the Cheltenham and the Bear of Rodborough Croquet Clubs. He was founder chairman of the Eastern Croquet Federation where he was instrumental in the creation of the Eastern Championships.

He has been a member of the Croquet Association Council for many years, with special responsibility for four of the season-long national tournaments. He is an examining referee and a qualified coach at all levels, being named 'Coach of the Year 1991'.

HOW TO USE THIS BOOK

The purpose of this book is to enable you to teach yourself association croquet. Association croquet is the official version of the game in almost all countries of the world where croquet is played. It is also the version recognised by the World Croquet Federation for international events. *Note:* The term 'garden croquet' is often used, e.g. 'garden croquet set'. This is *not* a different version of croquet. It only refers to the place where croquet is played.

If you follow each chapter carefully you will, by the end of the book, be able to play croquet sufficiently well not only to enjoy the game but also to appreciate some of the subtleties of tactical play that croquet possesses.

Chapter 1 introduces the game with a brief history, followed by an outline of the rules. Read this chapter, perhaps using some counters on a piece of paper to help understand the moves. Do not try to play on the lawn yet.

Chapter 2 describes the equipment used. If you have not yet bought a set this may help you to choose. If you have a set already, it will tell you about the equipment in it. Thus armed, the last item to get right before playing is the lawn. The standard layout is shown, followed by suggestions on layout for those who have unusually shaped or small lawns.

In Chapter 3, play commences. You learn how to hold a mallet and how to strike a ball. A game is described which helps you to practise this.

Chapter 4 is perhaps the most important in the book. It describes in depth, the shot which is unique to the game of croquet – the *two-ball shot*. Read the chapter carefully, then practise the shots on a lawn.

Having learned the mechanics of the game, Chapter 5 shows how to actually play a game. It covers how to start, where to place balls, and tactics. Chapter 6 describes how to finish. Read these chapters first, then try out the ideas on a lawn.

The remaining chapters of the book cover topics which can be read separately. Chapter 7 describes ways of scoring. It also shows a method by which better players can be handicapped to make games more even. Read this chapter only when the basic game has been mastered. Chapter 8 contains a comprehensive reference list of the rules of association croquet. A number of games other than association croquet can be played on a croquet lawn. Chapter 9 describes how to play some of them.

For those who wish to proceed further with croquet, the final chapter gives information on joining the Croquet Association (the CA) or a club. It also gives a selected list of further books on the game.

Acknowledgements

No teaching book can ever be entirely the work of only one person. A good teacher is someone who passes on to others the knowledge gained from his or her own mentors. To this is added the teacher's personal experience. The result is, hopefully, a continually widening circle of knowledge. I hope that this book will widen the circle a little further.

My sincere thanks to those who taught me and to the following people who have made a specific contribution to the book. To Michael and Claire Hearfield for trying out the ideas. To Allan Parker of Parkstone Croquet Club and Tom Anderson of Wrest Park Croquet Club for contributions to the history chapter. To Peter Dorke of Ludlow Croquet Club for proof-reading the draft. To Martin French of Ipswich Croquet Club for comments on the rules.

I would also like to thank the following for their help with the photographs: Worthing Croquet Club for the cover, Tom Anderson for the Beddows Cup, Charles Townsend for the loan of a croquet set and Ipswich Croquet Club for the loan of their lawns.

1

— WHAT IS CROQUET? —

——— A brief history of croquet ———

The following description appeared in an account of an early croquet tournament held in 1872 at Wimbledon at the All England Croquet Club:

'Near the village of Wimbledon, on the very brink of the railway that hurries you thither and then bears off the rest of the passengers towards Southampton, Bombay, Jamaica, or wherever they wish to go, are four acres of grassy land. These acres are laid out in three terraces, the one above the other, and on each terrace are four croquet grounds. From a croquet point of view these grounds are simply perfection. Each is forty yards by thirty . . . beautifully levelled, and the yellows and pinks and blues of the rolling balls are resplendent in the sunshine.

Croquet in the eyes of experts is not a mania, nor the imbecility of first or second childhood. It is a very fascinating and very difficult game, requiring nerve, judgement, unremitting attention, and a great physical nicety . . . and I think we may almost say already that it is the most absorbing game yet invented . . . Early on Tuesday certain strange mallets, with their owners, were collected together at the Waterloo station – flat mallets, cylindrical mallets, heavy mallets, light mallets – and soon the Wimbledon croquet ground began to fill . . .'

It seems that the habit of making fun of croquet in articles existed even then, despite an obviously serious tournament played on good lawns with good equipment. It was not until 1877 that the first lawn tennis championship was held at Wimbledon, yet within five years croquet had virtually been ousted by tennis.

Despite this setback, croquet was flourishing:

> 'Croquet is a game of very modern invention, and yet, in a few years it forced its way into such extraordinary popularity, that there is not a parish in the kingdom where the game is not known – scarcely a lawn, suitable or unsuitable, where the hoops were not to be seen; scarcely a house of any pretensions above those of the labourer's cottage, in whose entrance hall or passage the long white deal box, which tells of mallets and balls within, was not a prominent object.'

So commences the Rev J G Wood MA, FLS, writing in *The Boy's Modern Playmate – A Book of Sports, Games and Pastimes*, published in 1893.

Yet Cassell's *Book of Sports and Pastimes Illustrated*, published only three years later, starts its section on croquet thus:

> 'Never, probably, has there been a game so universally and thoroughly popular in Great Britain as croquet, and never was a popularity so rapidly achieved or so soon undermined and thrown into the shade when its zenith had once been achieved'.

So croquet has had its ups and downs. The Edwardian era was probably croquet's highest point in terms of widespread play, while its lowest was to be during and just after the Second World War. It could well be argued, however, that in terms of availability to all, and in international recognition, croquet today is more widely played than ever before. One croquet equipment manufacturer estimates that there are now between a quarter and half a million people playing croquet in the UK.

The origins of croquet

How did croquet start? Many sources quote the game of Pall Mall as its origin. This was a game played in a straight line with large hoops and a mallet looking like a golf club. It had only a slight resemblance to modern croquet. It is not even certain that there is any connection between the game and the present Pall Mall in London. References give a variation of spellings such as Pallemaille and Pele Mele.

The name 'croquet' would seem to indicate a French origin, but it is quite likely that it was chosen simply for the sound. Cassell's *New French Dictionary* gives the definition of croquet as 'a game or a crisp biscuit'. It is interesting that the sticks which are used to indicate extra turns in handicap croquet are called bisques. The dictionary also gives one definition of crochet as a 'hooked stick' (shepherds crook?) and the verb croquer 'to crunch together'. Nothing is known for certain though, and the mystery remains.

The first known reference to a game that resembled proper croquet came from Ireland in the early part of the nineteenth century. The following is an extract from *Notes on Croquet and Some Ancient Bat and Ball Games Related to It* by R C A Prior MD, FLS in 1872:

'As to its introduction into this country the meagre result of all the enquiries that I have been able to make is only this: that I learned from Mr Spratt, of 18 Brook Street, Hanover Square, that more than twenty years ago a Miss Macnaghten brought it to him as a game that had been lately introduced into Ireland, but which she had first seen on the continent . . .

Around 1850, John Jaques, a toy manufacturer, produced a croquet set and his firm has been doing so ever since. There were, however, other manufacturers and many variations were to be found. Some of these were quite bizarre. For example, in one version a four-way hoop was set in the middle of the lawn with a bell suspended in the middle which had to be rung to finish. The number of hoops varied from six to ten, with one or two pegs. Even today there is a version with nine hoops and two pegs which is played in some places in America.

The developing game

As the century progressed, so did croquet. Clubs and associations began to be formed and the game spread round the British empire and even to America. As so often happens when a game becomes more popular, dissent started to occur and several rival organisations were created. Each of these claimed to be the true representative of the sport. Worse than this, croquet became associated with immoral behaviour. In England it was rumoured that young ladies would knock their ball into the shrubbery and would disappear with a young gentleman to look for it! In America things were even worse with, in 1890, the city of Boston banning the game.

By 1882, croquet had been ousted from Wimbledon by tennis and was in decline. Its revival commenced just before the end of the century. The United All England Croquet Association (later to become the present Croquet Association) was formed and by the outbreak of the Great War there were 170 registered clubs. These were the Edwardian days, considered by many to be the golden era of croquet. However, the war brought about the closure of many clubs, some of them for ever.

After the war, in 1918, croquet continued at a lower level. Two significant events to occur were the introduction of the advanced rules game for top players, and today's six-hoop and one peg setting.

The most radical change however was the 'either ball' rule. Previously, the balls were played in sequence. This meant that a player always knew exactly which ball was to be played next by his or her opponent. This ball would be put into a distant corner. It was then very difficult for the opponent to score. The new rule meant that at the start of a turn players could choose either of their own two balls to play with, irrespective of the one played on the previous turn. This rule, which is played today, makes the game much less one-sided.

The Beddows Cup

A problem which arose before and after the First World War was the loss of prestigious cups due to their being won outright. Nowadays cups can be won for one year only, but in the past, a cup won on three or four occasions was the winner's to keep. Some players re-donated them but others did not. One who did not was a Miss D D Steel. Tom Anderson from Wrest Park Croquet Club tells the story of the Beddows Cup.

'The Beddows Cup was the trophy for the Open Championships until 1933. That year Miss D D Steel from Bedford Croquet Club won it for the fourth time and was allowed to keep it. This trophy then disappeared from view in the croquet world.

I re-discovered the cup in 1978. Reading a local newspaper, I noticed an entry in the classified ads columns: "Bedfordshire Croquet Cup for Sale". The vendor, I discovered, was a local small antique dealer who was moving away and "wanted the cup to remain in Bedfordshire".

The cup is solid silver with large handles, about three feet tall, with a velvet lined box to hold it. It is very ornate, having a laurel wreath and crossed mallets surmounting the lid. There is a relief of a croquet scene all round one side of the cup, depicting a gentleman playing croquet and two lady spectators standing by a tent.

After seeing the cup we began to search for its identity. Looking through old Croquet Association records, we were able to correlate

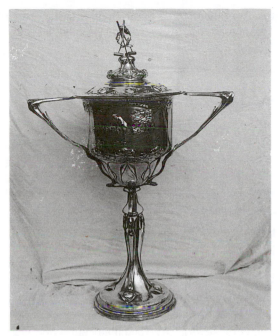

The Beddows Cup

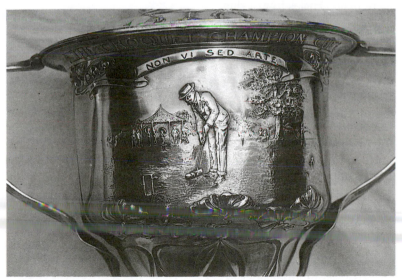

Detail from The Beddows Cup

the winners' names with those of the Beddows Cup. To avoid losing the cup again, possibly for ever, we purchased it, and have it to this day.'

The modern game

The Second World War saw an almost complete cessation of competitive croquet. It also resulted in the immediate or eventual closure of about half the clubs in the country. Picking itself up from this sorry state, the CA did what it could with what remained. By the 1950s, the major tournaments of the calendar were running well, and although there was not much growth, there was at least no deterioration.

The story from then to the present day has been one of a steady growth in popularity. Particularly satisfying has been the success of the CA in attracting sponsorship for major events, resulting in media attention which has helped to make the game more widely known.

Another success story has been the growth of new clubs. Thanks to efforts by the CA and regional croquet bodies, plus sterling work by bands of volunteers, several large and many small new clubs have been formed. Today it is rare for anyone not living in a remote rural area to be more than 30 miles from a club.

Recent years have also seen the emergence of expert young players. Although it is not true to say that they dominate totally, very many major events are now being won by teenagers.

Worldwide, croquet is co-ordinated by the World Croquet Federation. The rules of association croquet are the international rules used for the World Croquet Championships. These have been held since 1989. Croquet is widely played in Australia, New Zealand, South Africa, and the USA. It is also played to a lesser extent in Canada, France, Ireland, Italy, Japan, Spain, Sweden and Switzerland. Scotland, the Channel Islands, the Isle of Man and Wales have their own associations for administration, although they work closely with the English CA.

So croquet has come a long way in a relatively short time. Many things have changed, yet, again quoting from Cassell's book: 'It was the first successful attempt that had been made to invent an outdoor game in which both sexes could join on terms of equality, in which old and young could take part with equal chances . . .' These words are as true today as they were then.

──────── How to play croquet ────────

You may find it helpful to refer to fig. 1 throughout this section. *Note:* There is a glossary of terms at the end of the book.

The aim of the game

A croquet lawn is laid out with six hoops and one peg arranged as shown in fig. 1 on page 8. The object of the game is to get a ball through the hoops in the direction and order indicated. When a ball has passed through all hoops correctly, it can be made to strike the centre peg. It is then *pegged out* and has completed the game. The first player or pair to peg out both balls is the winner.

First principles

A game may be played by two people or four. Two play each other as 'singles', while four play in two opposing pairs as 'doubles'. There are four balls, each coloured differently. The usual four colours are blue, black, red and yellow. These colours will be used for describing play in this book. Sometimes you will see a set coloured brown, green, pink and white. These are called secondary colours and are often used when two games occupy the same lawn. Do not worry if your set has different colours. As long as you remember which player has which ball, the colour does not matter. Corresponding to the four balls are four coloured clips. These clips are placed on the top of the hoops to indicate which hoop each ball should pass through next. At the start of a game therefore, all clips will be placed on top of hoop one. As soon as a player successfully runs this hoop, he or she will move the correctly coloured clip to hoop two.

In singles, each player has two of the balls. It is conventional that the darker colours play the lighter. In this case therefore, blue/black plays red/yellow.

In doubles, each player has one ball and can only play with that ball during the match. However, there are not four individual opponents. The game is played with two pairs. Like doubles in tennis, the game is played as though each pair is a single unit, each individual in the pair playing his/her part as required.

The game starts with the toss of a coin. The winner/s can choose (a) to

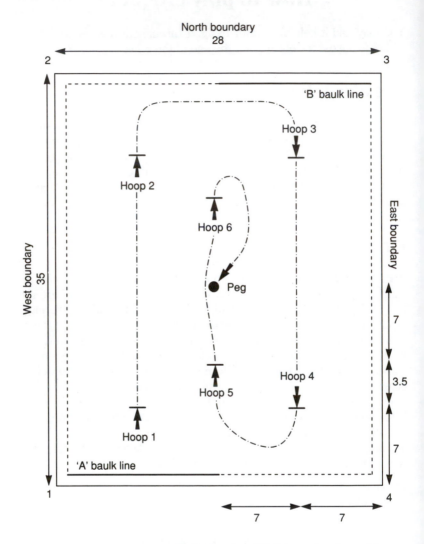

Fig. 1: The standard court

play first or second, or (b) what colours to play with. The loser/s therefore get whatever option is left. The winner will normally go for option (a) since there is usually no particular advantage in choosing colours.

A common misunderstanding should be corrected at this point. The peg will often have colours painted on it. This has *no* bearing whatsoever on the order of play.

Assume that the winner of the toss has chosen to go in first and that the loser has chosen red/yellow. Then either black or blue (in doubles, either the player of black or the player of blue) may play first. Assume black plays first. In the next turn the opponent(s) can play either red or yellow. Assume that it is red. Now blue must play next, followed by yellow. All four balls are now in play.

Having got all four balls into play, each side may opt to play the ball which is most advantageous. Thus blue/black may opt to play black for several turns in succession. (In doubles this would mean that one partner has several turns in succession.) Naturally no-one is allowed to strike a ball of the opposing side.

The starting point for each of the four balls is also shown in fig. 1. It is along one of the two lines marked 'A' baulk or 'B' baulk. Note that the baulk lines only extend half-way across the court. Fig. 2 shows the location of the line more clearly. The choice of baulk line and the position along it is made by the player. (It might appear logical at this stage always to choose baulk 'A', which is of course nearer to hoop one. However, later chapters show that the choice of baulk 'B' is often made for sound tactical reasons.)

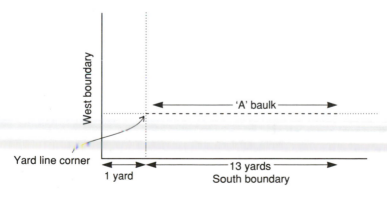

Fig. 2: The 'A' baulk line

Extra shots

The sections which follow, and others later in the book, describe various movements of mallets and balls. In order to avoid confusion it is important to distinguish between two quite separate movements: your mallet *striking* your ball, and a ball, while travelling across the court, *hitting* another. In this book therefore, strike, striking, etc. will mean your mallet striking your ball and hit, hitting, etc. will mean balls hitting each other.

If the only thing that could be done in croquet was to take it in turns to try to strike your ball through a series of hoops in sequence, the game would be trivial. Fortunately there are a number of ways in which your turn can be extended.

In snooker an extra shot is gained by potting a ball. Similarly, in croquet an extra shot is gained by striking your ball so that it passes through a hoop. This is called *running a hoop* or *scoring a hoop*. It has already been noted that each of your two balls (or in doubles, each partner's ball) must pass once through every hoop as shown in fig. 1. The diagram shows clearly that it might just be possible with a very accurate shot to run, say, hoop one, then with your extra shot, run hoop two. It would not be possible, however, to do the same between hoops two and three. More is therefore needed if progress is desired past hoop two within the same turn.

The game is extended still further by giving *two* extra shots if you are able to strike your ball so that it hits another. The way that these two extra shots are played is described below.

First extra shot

When your ball hits another, you pick up your ball and place it in contact with the ball that it has just hit. Then you strike your ball (not both) so that both balls move. The way that your ball is placed and the way that it is struck by your mallet determines how far and in what direction each ball will travel. Chapter 4 explains in detail how to do this.

Second extra shot

You then have one more shot with your ball only. With this shot you can either run a hoop or hit another ball.

Making a break

From the start (very first stroke) of your turn, you are allowed, if you wish, to hit each of the other three balls and place your ball next to it (as described above) once, without running a hoop. If you have hit all three and do not then run a hoop with your last extra shot, your turn must end. As soon as you run a hoop, however, you are once more allowed to hit all of the other balls. Irrespective of the way that this turn finishes, on your next turn, you can once again hit each of the other three balls.

So, with care and skill, it is possible to play so that the hitting of other balls, the subsequent striking of two balls placed together and the running of hoops, all combine to produce a situation in which many hoops can be run in a single turn. The tactics and skill required to make breaks in this way are what makes croquet such an interesting game. Croquet is not meant to be played in a negative fashion, concentrating solely on the destruction of your opponent. Played like that, it becomes boring. Played with prudent aggression and style, the game becomes an exciting challenge, with the rewards of a well-fought contest.

Finishing

A game is finished when both balls of a player or pair have run all of the hoops and then hit the peg. This may be done by hitting the peg with each ball in two separate turns. A better way, however, is to have your other ball (in doubles, your partner's ball) near the peg. Then, after the last hoop has been run, arrange your game so that you can hit your other ball. Your ball is picked up, and placed in contact with your other ball. With the first extra shot, cause your other ball to hit the peg. With the second, hit the peg with your own ball.

A pegged out ball is removed from the game, so if for some reason only one ball is pegged out, only the other ball can be played in subsequent turns (in doubles this means that only the player of the remaining ball can play). Chapter 6 describes in detail how to finish a game.

Other rules

Out of court

In the shot where you put your ball against the one you have just hit, neither ball must go out of court. If this happens the turn ends and any ball that went off is replaced on the yard line (see below). *Note:* In all other shots where a ball goes out of court, the ball is replaced on the yard line without any penalty.

There is an imaginary line one yard in from the boundary and parallel to it. It is on this line that balls are replaced if they go out of court. Fig. 1 shows the yard line. If a ball goes out of court within one yard of a corner, it is replaced on the yard line corner. Fig. 2 shows a yard line corner.

A ball passes out of court if any part of it touches or crosses the inside edge of the court boundary line. Fig. 3 shows this.

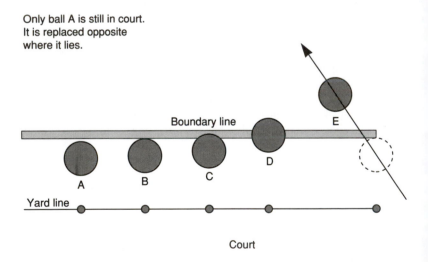

Balls B, C, D and E are out.
They are replaced at the point marked with a dot.
Note particularly ball E.
This was travelling at an angle,
and is replaced opposite the exact point where it went out.

Only ball A is still in court.
It is replaced opposite
where it lies.

Boundary line

E

D

A   B   C

Yard line

Court

Fig. 3: When a ball is out of court

Running a hoop

A ball has run a hoop, and scores a hoop point, when it passes through the correct hoop in the correct direction. The part of the hoop which faces the striker as he or she is about to run the hoop is called the *playing side*. A ball starts to run a hoop when its leading edge can be seen beyond the hoop on the non-playing side, when looking at the hoop side-on. A ball completes the running of a hoop when its trailing edge passes beyond the playing side and cannot be seen when looking at the hoop side-on. A ball may run a hoop in more than one turn, that is, having started to run in one turn, it can complete in another.

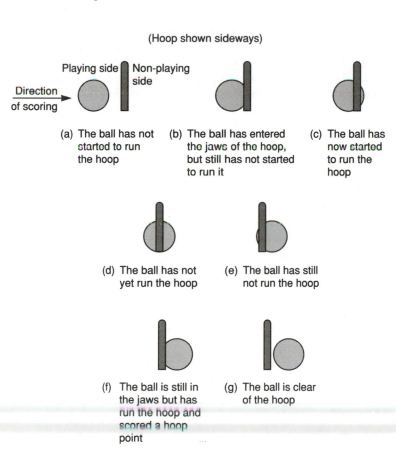

(Hoop shown sideways)

Playing side | Non-playing side

Direction of scoring

(a) The ball has not started to run the hoop

(b) The ball has entered the jaws of the hoop, but still has not started to run it

(c) The ball has now started to run the hoop

(d) The ball has not yet run the hoop

(e) The ball has still not run the hoop

(f) The ball is still in the jaws but has run the hoop and scored a hoop point

(g) The ball is clear of the hoop

Fig. 4: Scoring a hoop point

Fig. 4 on page 13 illustrates the scoring of a hoop point.

A ball other than your ball can be made to score its hoop; for example by sending it through its hoop when you hit it with your ball. This is called peeling. The clip for the peeled ball is moved to the next hoop for that ball.

Hitting the peg

Only a ball which has run all of its hoops can hit and score the peg or cause another ball to hit the peg. There is no penalty for hitting the peg with a ball which has not run all of its hoops.

Fig. 1 shows that six hoops are run in a single direction by each ball, plus one peg point for each ball, making a total of 14 points per player or pair of players. This is the most suitable version for garden croquet. However, it is possible to make a longer game by running the hoops again, but in the opposite direction. This longer game is described in Chapter 7.

Metrication

Croquet has not yet moved into metres and centimetres. To help those who do not use imperial measurements, a metric conversion of standard measurements is given in brackets. For example, the correct diameter of a ball is 3⅝ inches (92mm). In the case of many of the exercises, a measure has been used simply for convenience (for example, 'put the balls a yard apart'). In these exercises, for 'yard' read 'metre', 'foot' read '300mm', 'inch' read '25mm'.

Misunderstandings in croquet

One of the intentions of this book is to dispel the misunderstandings that surround croquet. The following are *not* true.

'Oh that's the game where you put your foot on the ball.' It is not, this is not allowed.

'It's a game played by old ladies.' Yes it is, but it is also played by women (and men) of all ages.

'Croquet is an elitist game.' No it is not, it is played by people from all walks of life.

'Ah yes, that's where you play with flamingoes for mallets.' If Lewis Carroll could have known the trouble he would cause, he would have never written that part!

'The idea of croquet is to send your opponent's ball into the shrubbery.' Not true, it is a fault to send a ball out of court.

'Croquet is a vicious sport.' This comes from the misconception that croquet is all about separating your opponent.

No doubt you will have heard others, plus all sorts of strange ideas on how to play. Well, there is only one set of rules in this country, and they are taught in this book – so please read on!

2

EQUIPMENT AND LAWNS

—————— Equipment ——————

Mallets

It is possible to play with only one mallet, all sharing, but preferably each player should have his or her own. Shapes and sizes vary, but a typical mallet will have these characteristics:

- Weight about three pounds (1.4kg)
- Shaft length about one yard (0.9m)
- Head length about 9–12 inches (225–300mm).

For children, shafts may be shorter, but the weight should be the same.

Some mallets have round heads, some square. There is no advantage of one over the other, it is merely personal preference. Some mallets are even made of metal with plastic ends.

Care of mallets

Most garden set mallets are made entirely of wood. A regular coating of protective varnish will help preserve the mallet from damp. If the mallet gets wet, do not dry it too quickly. Store it in a cool dry place, either flat in a box, or hanging from a hook by the head. Do not leave it leaning against a wall as the handle may warp. If the mallet has a metal band at the ends, make sure that it does not protrude and damage the balls (or people).

Balls

These may be of compound, plastic or, occasionally, wood. They should weigh about one pound (454g) and have a diameter of 3⅝ inches (92mm).

Care of balls

If the balls are of wood, the same care should be taken as for mallets except that paint of the appropriate colour is used instead of varnish. No special care need be taken with compound or plastic balls as far as normal use is concerned.

Underweight mallets and balls

If your croquet set is of very light construction, an enjoyable game of croquet can still be had, but some care needs to be taken. Very hard shots on heavy lawns should be avoided as there is a danger of breaking the mallet shaft.

Some croquet strokes (see Chapter 4) may not be possible with an underweight croquet set. In particular:

- With light mallets (less than 2lbs) roll strokes will be difficult.
- With light balls (less than ¾lb) stop shots will be difficult.
- With light balls *and* light mallets, croquet strokes in general may not bchave exactly as predicted in this book.

Clips

Where provided these should be used as described in this book. If they are not provided, wooden clothes pegs painted the appropriate colours will work well.

Flags and corner pegs

These are not essential to a game, but if your set has them, fig. 35 on page 105 shows where they should be placed.

Hoops and peg

The best hoops are those of sturdy metal construction, using five-eighths of an inch diameter uprights and a welded square top. These are, however, expensive and less robust hoops may have to suffice. If your hoops are of the thin wire variety, they will work well for normal play but very hard shots where the ball hits the hoop should be avoided as damage can result.

If you have a hoop with a blue painted top, make this the first hoop. If you have a hoop with a red painted top, make this the last hoop. Any other colours can be ignored.

Setting the hoops

Unless the ground is soft, it is better to make pilot holes first with a spike. Use a wooden mallet to drive the hoops and the peg into the ground. If you do not have one, place an old piece of wood on top of the hoop and strike that. Make slight adjustments to the width of a hoop by packing the sides of the holes with grass cuttings or earth. The width of the hoops should be a quarter of an inch (6 mm) wider than the balls. Check that all the balls are the same diameter. If they are not, use the widest ball for setting the hoops.

Croquet sets

Many sports shops sell croquet sets, although you will probably need to go to a larger shop to obtain the better quality sets. Often, the national associations for each country (see Appendix 1) will sell croquet equipment. The first photograph in the colour plate section shows a middle-of-the-range croquet set. Such a set will sell for around £175. Simpler sets are available at around £100. If you want a complete set of championship standard equipment, it could cost you around £1000.

Appendix 2 on page 129 provides a list of manufacturers of croquet equipment around the world.

--------------------------------- **Lawns** ---------------------------------

The ideal lawn is perfectly flat, closely cut and a symmetrical rectangle with the dimensions shown in fig. 1. Only a lucky few with big gardens can hope to approach the ideal, but good play is still possible on small, and even oddly-shaped lawns.

These simple guidelines will improve playing conditions considerably:

- Cut the grass reasonably short. Bowling green standard is normally not possible but playing on grass an inch long is difficult and unpredictable. Do not cut your lawn *too* short if it is bumpy or on a big slope. If you do so, it will be very difficult to control the direction of the balls.

- Clear the lawn of any huge weeds, especially near hoops. Large weeds will often deflect a ball.
- If possible, move hoops occasionally to even out wear on the grass.

Small and odd-shaped lawns

The regulation dimensions of 35 by 28 yards (32 by 25.6 metres) represent a large lawn. This is about the size of two tennis courts, but a perfectly satisfactory game can be had on a much smaller area. Even a piece of ground 10 by 5 yards (9 by 4.5 metres) will do, although there are obviously very few really difficult shots on something that small. Anything smaller than this is not really practical for six hoops. If this is all that is available, set out three hoops in a triangle with the peg in the middle, and run them twice, going through in the opposite direction the second time.

The measurements given in fig. 1 should be reduced in the same ratio as the lawn. So half length or width equals half the measurement.

Irrespective of the size of the lawn, keep the yard line at one yard. This is so that play within the yard line area can take place normally. However, if you only have the tiny lawn with three hoops mentioned above, you could reduce the yard line to half a yard.

Strange-shaped lawns can make for some very interesting games! Fig. 5 on page 20 gives a few suggestions for some common shapes. Note that in each case the order and direction of hoops is kept similar to the standard layout.

If you have a tree or other obstruction in the lawn, make a local rule that there is a free movement of balls if your swing is impeded by the tree. However, such movement must not give an advantage. For example, you should not have a clear shot at a ball if none existed from the original position. Also, any ball hitting the tree and bouncing off is played where it lies (subject to the swing rule just given).

If you have a small flower bed or similar in the middle of the lawn, treat this as a boundary in the same way as the normal boundary, i.e. your turn ends if you go over the edge.

So, you now have a lawn and a croquet set plus a general idea of the game. It's time to start striking a ball.

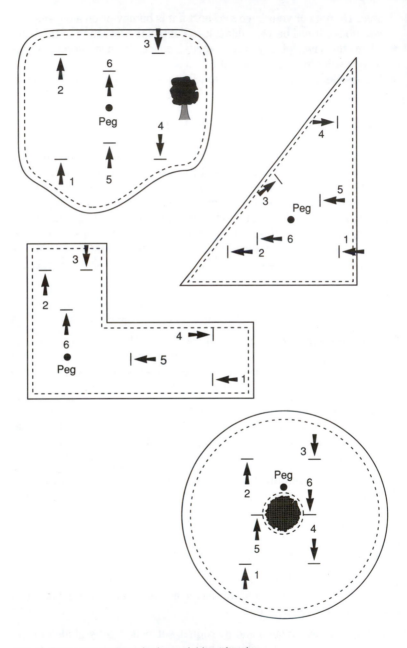

Fig. 5: Some non-rectangular lawns laid out for play

3

– STRIKING THE BALL –

——— Holding your mallet ———

Stance

There are two main ways to stand when taking a shot. These are called the centre and the side styles.

In the centre style, which is the most common, you face the ball directly and in line with the direction in which you intend to send the ball, standing with each foot equally spaced either side of the ball. You then swing the mallet between your legs.

In the side style, you still face the direction in which you intend to send the ball, but stand to one side of the ball. You either keep your feet together, or place one slightly in front of the other – whichever feels most comfortable. Your mallet is swung parallel to the side of your body. Normally, right-handed players would play to the right and left-handed players to the left but the mallet may be swung from either side – the choice is personal.

There are other, less common styles. The mallet can be held and played like a golf putter or a cricket bat. A few players find this suits them but it is unusual.

Colla Steward demonstrates the side style in photograph 2 in the colour section, while photographs 3–5 all show centre style, but with different grips (see page 22). Notice in each picture how the player is facing along the line of strike.

Grip

There is no 'perfect' way of holding a mallet. The important thing is to find a grip which suits you. This section describes the most common types of grip. It is recommended that you experiment with them to find the most suitable.

The standard grip

Photograph 2 in the colour section shows the so-called standard grip. It *is* a very common grip, but there is no such thing as a standard way of holding a mallet. Celia has her left hand at the top of the mallet and her right hand about a foot down the shaft. Notice that she is holding her left thumb over the top of the shaft, and her right index finger is pointing down the shaft. It is not essential to do this, but many players who use the standard grip do so because they feel that it helps them swing the mallet more accurately. You should hold the mallet in a way that feels comfortable for you.

In photograph 3, the author, who is a left-handed player, is also using a standard grip, but his hands are held much closer together. He uses the index finger for guidance, but not the thumb. Having the hands closer together helps the arms swing as a single unit, but makes the mallet more difficult to control.

The Irish grip

1991 World Champion John Walters is using the Irish grip in photograph 4. This grip is good for balancing the arms and is extremely accurate when played well. It does, however, take a lot of getting used to, and places a lot of strain on the wrists. If you find that you like this style, do not play too much croquet at first, or your wrists will complain!

The Solomon grip

Named after John Solomon, a champion player, the Solomon grip is demonstrated by Celia Pearce in photograph 5. As you can see from Celia's arms, this is a very symmetrical grip. It is frequently used by players who adopt method two of striking the ball (see page 26). Like the Irish grip, the Solomon needs practice and can be hard on the wrists.

Other grips

Many players adopt grips which are combinations of the above. Try the exercises below, and find out which suits you best.

EXERCISES

1 Experiment with centre and side stances and see which feels the best for you. Hit a ball to get the feel of the stance but don't worry about what happens to the ball, concentrate only on the stance.

2 Experiment with the different grips and see which feels the best for you. Hit a ball to get the feel of the grip but don't worry about what happens to the ball, concentrate only on the grip. Be aware that those grips which have the hands close together will often need a longer time to get used to than those with the hands further apart. Don't fix on a grip for all time at this stage, but do give the one that you choose time to work.

– Striking the ball to hit another ball –

Although the ability to send a ball in the required direction is only part of croquet, it is a vitally important part. If you do not hit another ball or run a hoop, you will not get any more shots and your turn ends.

To hit another ball, imagine a piece of string joining the centre of your ball with the centre of the one you want to hit. Now extend that string beyond the balls. Stand well back from your ball, facing both, and walk slowly towards your ball along the imaginary string. Stop about a foot from your ball and take stance (centre or side). The correct positions are shown on page 24. If you look ahead, you should be looking directly at the other ball. If you look down you should be looking straight at your ball. Your mallet should be resting lightly on the ground, directly facing the ball in the direction in which you want to send it.

This procedure is called *stalking the ball*. Its purpose is to ensure that your body is correctly placed so you are facing in the same direction as the line formed by the imaginary string.

The exact distance to stand behind the ball will come with practice. If you are tending to strike your ball with the bottom of your mallet, you may be too far back. If your ball jumps in the air when you strike it, you may be too close (sometimes this happens if you lean forward just as you go to strike your ball).

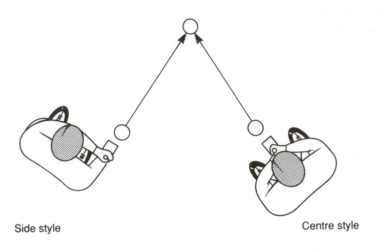

Side style   Centre style

Fig. 6: Taking your stance

Playing the shot (1)

Having taken the correct stance, line up your shot. This can best be done by taking a few practice swings over the top of the ball. Then rest your mallet on the ground, directly behind your ball and compose yourself for the shot.

The actual shot can be split into three parts: the backswing, striking the ball and the follow-through.

The backswing

It is during the backswing that you are lining up your mallet to strike your ball. Your backswing should therefore be sufficient to allow you to do this. If you only take a very short backswing, you are likely to jerk the mallet off line. There is no 'correct' amount of backswing but your mallet head should travel about a yard before hitting the ball for a fairly firm shot. This travel can be reduced for shots that are less forceful but there should always be some swing. In photograph 6 in the colour section, the author is attempting to strike his ball onto the peg. Notice the amount of backswing used, and his concentration on the ball.

The strike

Don't force the mallet to change direction at the end of the backswing.
Let it change naturally. The secret of a good swing is to 'let the mallet do
the work'. If you find that hitting the ball is an effort, you are not letting
the mallet work for you. If you swing sweetly, you will strike the ball
sweetly. In photograph 7, the ball has just been struck. Note that the
centre of the mallet head has struck the ball.

The follow-through

Just as the backswing is important in getting the mallet on the right line,
so the follow-through is important in keeping it there. Your mallet should
be allowed to stop moving naturally – do not force it to do so.

Photograph 8 shows the ball striking the peg, but the striker is not
looking at the ball. This is because his follow-through is only just
finishing. Note the position of the mallet and the striker's head.

An essential ingredient of any good shot is to keep your eye on the ball
during the backswing and strike. In fact it is fairly easy to watch the ball at
this stage, but it is the most natural thing in the world to follow the mallet
head up after the strike to see where your ball is going. The most natural,
and totally wrong! Keep your eyes on the spot where the ball was until
the follow-through is complete. By doing this, you will keep your mallet
on the right line. Photographs 6–8 illustrate this point.

Throughout the three parts of the shot there is a common thread – keep
it smooth. Watch any player of any sport where a ball is struck. The best
shots seem to be played without effort. The same applies to croquet.

Some other hints

Do . . .

- Practise your swing before striking your ball.

- Make sure that you are facing the ball. Your practice swings should
  help. Imagine that you have struck your ball and follow the line of your
  swing, to see where the ball would go.

- Stand firmly but not stiffly.

- Move the whole of your arms as a single unit. Swing from the
  shoulders, not the wrists.

- Keep an even, firm but not tense grip with both hands.

Don't . . .

- Stand stiffly upright with your arms held rigidly down, making a sort of lunge at the ball. This is a common and understandable fault with beginners because there is a lot to remember.

- Move or lean forward before your follow-through is over. A symptom of this happening is that your ball jumps in the air when you hit it. Be careful though, as long clumps of grass can give the same effect.

- Twist your wrists.

- Grip more firmly with one hand than the other.

- 'Bounce' as you swing through. This is caused by excessive bending of the knees as you swing.

Playing the shot (2)

This is an alternative method of playing the shot. It is one adopted by many of the top young players. It is extremely accurate when played properly, but many find it more difficult to execute than the method described above.

Having stalked the ball and taken the correct stance, line up your shot by taking practice swings over the top of the ball. When you have the line correct, drop your mallet on the final backswing and strike the ball. The secret is to play the final swing which actually strikes the ball in exactly the same way as the practice swings.

The comments made in the previous section regarding backswing, the strike and follow-through apply equally to this method of play. So also does the remark about a smooth shot.

Keeping your eyes on the ball is also as vital, but more difficult because you do not have that period when the mallet is static behind the ball in which to compose yourself.

EXERCISES

For each exercise, try both methods of playing the shot to see which suits you best.

1 From one yard away, make your ball hit another.

2 From five yards away, make your ball hit another.

You can consider yourself successful if you can regularly:

- For 1: hit the ball nine times out of ten.
- For 2: hit the ball five times out of ten.

—— Striking the ball to run a hoop ——

Much of what has been said about hitting another ball applies when attempting to run a hoop. There are, however, a couple of extra points to consider.

Even when directly in front of a hoop, you must be very accurate with your shot, since the gap is only a little wider than your ball. When you are at an angle that gap becomes very small indeed. So lining up and stalking the ball are vital. When directly in front of a hoop, you naturally aim for the centre of the gap. When you are making an attempt from an angle, your aiming point moves towards one of the hoop uprights. If your shot is from the right of the hoop, the aiming point moves to the left and vice-versa. Fig. 7 illustrates this. As shots become more angled, the aiming point will move further across. Eventually, you will find yourself aiming directly at an upright. You have then reached the limit beyond which it is not possible to run the hoop.

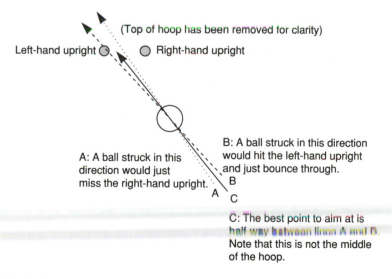

(Top of hoop has been removed for clarity)

Left-hand upright   Right-hand upright

B: A ball struck in this direction would hit the left-hand upright and just bounce through.

A: A ball struck in this direction would just miss the right-hand upright.

B

A   C

C: The best point to aim at is half way between lines A and B. Note that this is not the middle of the hoop.

Fig. 7: The aiming point for an angled hoop

The comments previously made about keeping your eye on the ball hold here as well. The temptation to look up immediately to see if you have successfully run the hoop is great. Resist it, you will know soon enough!

Photograph 9 in the colour section illustrates the technique of hoop running.

EXERCISES

For each exercise, try both methods of playing the shot to see which suits you best.

1 From one foot away and directly in front, make your ball run the hoop.

2 From one foot away and six inches to the side, make your ball run the hoop.

You can consider yourself successful if you can regularly:

- For 1: run the hoop nine times out of ten.
- For 2: run the hoop seven times out of ten.

Strength of shot

You have now seen how to strike your ball, either to hit another or to run a hoop. This section considers how hard you should play the shot.

Against another ball

You will recall from the description given in Chapter 1 that if you hit another ball with your own, you lift your ball and place it in contact with the ball you have hit. You can then play a shot which sends both balls in the required direction.

The ball that your ball hit in the first instance will have moved to a new position. Exactly where that new position is will be determined by the strength and angle with which your ball has hit it.

For example, suppose that you want to run a particular hoop. Your ball is directly behind (a few inches) the other ball, in line for your hoop, which is three yards away. If you only hit the other ball gently, the two-ball shot which follows (you will recall from Chapter 1 that you have two strokes, so you will be using one to get in front of the hoop and the other to run it) will take place nearly three yards from the hoop. If, however, you hit the other ball so that it travels the three yards to the hoop, your two shots take place right next to the hoop.

If the ball that you are going to hit with yours is very close to your own, it should be possible not only to hit it in a straight line but also (if needed) off-centre, so that it travels at an angle. Very close means no more than a couple of feet away.

Through a hoop

There will often be a ball waiting at the other side of your hoop. This ball will be used to continue your break when you have run the hoop. Chapter 4 shows how to put that ball there, in readiness, before you run the hoop. The strength with which you run the hoop will depend on the position of that ball.

If you are running the hoop from an angle, you will need to use more force than you would for a straight shot at the same distance because some of the energy is lost as the ball hits the hoop and bounces off. Care is needed, though, because the harder you strike a shot, the less accurate you tend to become.

Take particular care when your ball is very close to the hoop. It is not a fault to hit the hoop with your ball, nor is it a fault if you simply strike the hoop with your mallet. However, it *is* a fault and your turn ends if you 'crush' your ball against the hoop with your mallet. A crush occurs when the mallet strikes the ball in the direction of the hoop or peg without any room for follow-through. This is avoided by striking the ball away from the obstruction, allowing for free movement. Although a crush seems difficult to judge, it is usually fairly obvious to you as the striker. You are honour bound to admit the fault, replace the balls to where they were before the fault, and end your turn.

One useful tactic when your ball is close to the hoop is to give the ball a little flick with your mallet. Your mallet will then stop quickly and will not crush your ball.

EXERCISES

1   From one foot away, strike your ball so that it hits another, causing it to move for three yards in a straight line.

2   From one foot away, run a hoop and pass through by one yard.

3   From one foot away, run a hoop and pass through by three yards.

You can consider yourself successful if you can regularly:

- For 1: get the ball within two feet of where you want it.
- For 2: get the ball within one foot of where you want it.
- For 3: get the ball within one yard of where you want it.

Golf croquet

Despite its name this game is neither golf nor croquet! It is a simple game which is ideally suited to learning the skills which are described in this chapter, since nothing further is required other than a few simple tactics. It can be played with two players having two balls, four players with a ball each, or four players as two pairs. A turn is one single strike of your ball – there are no extra strokes in golf croquet. With that stroke you can do one of three things (occasionally you can do two of them in the same shot):

- Run a hoop (see law 3).

- Hit another ball.

- Take position, for example to run a hoop next time.

Balls are played in rotation (see law 8). If four people are playing, this means that each person has one shot in turn. If two are playing then players alternate both turns and balls, i.e. player A plays blue, player B plays red, player A plays black, player B plays yellow, etc.

The aim of the game

A game starts by spinning a coin. The winner chooses to go first or second, or colours, in the same way as association croquet. Each ball must be played into the game from anywhere on the 'B' baulk only. As soon as one ball has run a hoop, all players move on to contest the next one. A ball has to completely run a hoop in one turn. If it sticks, it has to come back (*Note:* this is *not* the same rule as association croquet). The exception to this rule is if your ball is knocked there by an opponent (not a partner). In this case you can run next turn (if it is still there). Each hoop scores one point. The winner is the one with the most points after all hoops have been run.

Rules of golf croquet

1   The contest is for six hoops, starting with hoop one and finishing with hoop six in the order shown in fig. 1 on page 8.

2   Each player has only one shot per turn. Play is strictly in sequence (see law 8). The shot may be used to (a) take position, (b) knock another ball out of the way or (c) run a hoop.

3   A ball runs a hoop in the same way as in association croquet (shown in fig. 4 on page 13). Unlike association croquet, if a ball starts to run a hoop but does not complete the running, i.e. it sticks in the jaws, it cannot score in the next stroke and must come back to try again. *Exception:* if the ball is placed there by an opponent it can run the hoop next turn.

4   When a ball runs a hoop, one point is scored for that ball's side and everyone moves on to the next hoop. *Note:* only *one* ball scores the hoop, not all.

5   There are six hoops, thus six points. When a player or side reaches an unbeatable score, i.e. scores four points, the game finishes and that player is the winner. If the score is three points each after the sixth hoop, continue (from where the balls lie) back to hoop one as a decider.

6   The game starts from anywhere along the 'B' baulk.

7   Any ball which goes out of court or into the yard line area is replaced one yard inside the boundary line from the point where it went off.

8   The normal sequence of play is blue, red, black, yellow. For second colour sets, the order is green, pink, brown, white. For other coloured sets, decide before playing.

9   The peg plays no part in the game except as an obstruction.

10   The game described is a short version. For a longer version see Chapter 7.

11   If two hoops are run in the same stroke, the striker scores two points and the game moves on two hoops.

12   Players must all contest the same hoop. A player is not allowed to assume that a hoop will be scored and so place his or her ball in advance for the next hoop.

13   If a player plays out of sequence, all balls are replaced and the correct player plays.

14   If a player plays a wrong ball, all balls are replaced and the correct ball is played.

Basic tactics

- Remember that golf croquet is a sequence game. Thus if you are playing red and cannot run the hoop, then black is the danger ball as black plays next (see law 8). The blue ball is less of a threat, but remember that black could hit yellow out of the way and yellow is the ball which precedes blue.

- When you are hitting balls out of the way, you may be able to do so in a way which puts your ball in front of the hoop.

- Instead of hitting an opponent ball, you can sometimes prevent a shot by putting your ball in the opponent's way.

- You can sometimes hit your partner ball and knock it in front of the hoop.

- If you are behind a hoop, you can block an opponent by jamming your ball in the hoop. Remember that you must clear the hoop in order to run it yourself.

4

— TWO-BALL SHOTS —

- The importance of the two-ball shot -

In Chapter 1, a two-ball shot was described as follows: *When your ball hits another, you pick up your ball and place it in contact with the ball that it has just hit. Then you strike your ball (not both) so that both balls move. The way that your ball is placed and the way that it is struck by your mallet determines how far and in what direction each ball will travel.*

Before the two-ball shot is explained more fully, it may be helpful to introduce a few croquet terms which describe this sequence. The hitting of another ball with your own is called a *roquet*, and the movement of the ball that you have hit is called a *rush*. The first extra shot – striking the two balls when placed together – is called the *croquet stroke* or *taking croquet* and the second extra shot is called the *continuation stroke*. Because these terms will be used a lot in this chapter, they are listed below so that you can refer to them easily. A full list of terms is included at the end of the book.

Roquet	– hitting another ball with your own.
The roqueted ball	– the ball that you have just hit. *Note:* when you play the croquet stroke, this ball becomes the croqueted ball.
Rush	– the movement of the roqueted ball when your ball hits it.
Croquet stroke (also **taking croquet**)	– striking your ball when it has been placed in contact with the roqueted ball.
The croqueted ball	– the other ball (not your ball) in a croquet stroke. *Note:* before taking croquet, this ball was called the roqueted ball.

Continuation stroke   – the extra shot that you have with your ball after a croquet stroke.

Although many sports require the accurate striking of the player's ball, and, in some cases, the subsequent hitting of others, it is only croquet that requires the accurate movement of *two* balls in a single stroke (in snooker it is a foul shot to move a ball that is touched by the cue ball).

The croquet stroke not only sets croquet apart from other stationary ball sports, it can truly be said to be central to the game. To strike one ball through a hoop requires skill, but to move two balls at the same time *and* position them with accuracy is much more challenging. A croquet player who can hit accurately will be quite successful, as will one with a good grasp of tactics. The player who can also play good croquet strokes will be formidable indeed. The croquet stroke is so important, this chapter is devoted almost completely to it.

It has to be said that croquet shots are easier to describe than to do. While there are a few lucky 'naturals' at the game, most of us mortals have to try very hard to make croquet shots work. So do not be surprised or disillusioned if things seem to go badly at first. Keep at it! It takes time but suddenly it will all click into place and you will start to play well.

First, a look at what leads to a croquet shot – the roquet.

Roquets and rushes

To be able to take croquet, you must make a roquet – i.e. hit another ball (see page 23). Note, though, that you take croquet from where you have rushed the roqueted ball (i.e., when it has stopped moving), not from where you originally hit it. Fig. 8 shows this.

This means that the rush is important in itself, not just something that happens as a result of making a roquet. With skill and planning you may be able to rush a ball to a part of the lawn where it will be much more useful than in its present position. The next chapter shows some of these useful positions.

EXERCISES

1   With your ball one foot away from another, roquet and rush the other ball for three yards in a straight line.

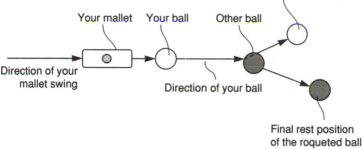

Fig. 8: Making a roquet

2 With your ball one foot away from another, roquet and rush the other ball for ten yards in a straight line.

3 With your ball one foot away from another, roquet and rush the other ball for one yard at an angle like that in fig. 8.

You will have grasped the idea if you can regularly:

- For 1: get the rushed ball within two feet of where you want it.
- For 2: get the rushed ball within three yards of where you want it.
- For 3: get the rushed ball within one foot of where you want it.

──────── The croquet stroke ────────

Definition

A croquet stroke is played by first placing your ball in contact with the roqueted ball, then striking your ball so that both move. Fig. 9 illustrates a typical croquet stroke.

You can see from fig. 9 over the page that the two balls move off in different directions. Why? Well, it all depends on the direction in which you strike your ball. Suppose that the croqueted ball had not been there in fig. 9. Your ball would naturally have travelled in the same direction that you struck it. The croqueted ball *is* there, however, so that some of

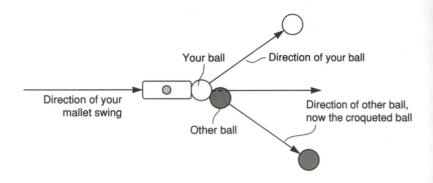

Fig. 9: A croquet stroke

the energy put into striking your ball passes through to the other one (this is why they have to be in contact – if they are not the shot does not work properly).

Prediction

Can you then predict where the balls will go? Yes you can.

The croqueted ball will travel along a line drawn through the centre of both balls. It will also travel at an angle from the line of your mallet swing. Your ball will travel at the same angle in the other direction. In other words, if the croqueted ball moves away at 20 degrees to the left, then your ball will move away at 20 degrees to the right.

'Very interesting', you say, 'but what does it mean?'

If fig. 9 is redrawn as fig. 10 and some lines are added, things will be clearer.

The movement of the croqueted ball is the easiest to predict. It is *always* going to travel along line A in fig. 10. So imagine this line on the lawn, then place your ball behind the other and on that line. Fig. 11 (opposite) shows how to choose two different directions.

To predict the direction of *your* ball requires more care. Look at fig. 10. The croqueted ball travels along line A. Your ball travels along line C. Your mallet swings along line B. So you are aiming at half the angle

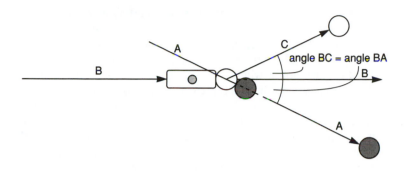

Fig. 10: A croquet stroke showing angles

To send the croqueted ball towards X, place your ball here

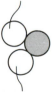

Note that as long as the croqueted ball *does* move, it will go towards X or Y irrespective of the direction in which your mallet swings

To send the croqueted ball towards Y, place your ball here

Fig. 11: Lining up the croqueted ball

between lines A and C. If you want to get technical the angle between lines A and C is twice that between lines A and B or between lines B and C.

But there is an easier way!

Execution

By repeating fig. 10 as fig. 12 and this time putting in another line (D) which joins the two balls after they have moved, you can see that line B (the one you swing your mallet along) crosses line D exactly halfway between the two balls. So you don't have to worry about angles unless you want to. Just look at where you want the two balls to go and *aim half way between them.* You can see this clearly in photograph 10 in the colour section. Celia wishes to place red in front of her hoop (on her left), and yellow behind it. In photograph 11, she has achieved this. If you compare the ball positions in 11 with the position of Celia in 10, you will see that she plays her croquet stroke by aiming midway between where she wants the two balls to go, i.e. just to her right of the hoop. Notice in 11 how Celia is carefully lining up the hoop stroke before taking her stance.

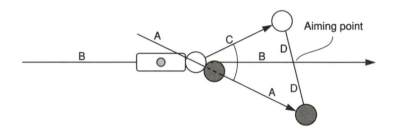

Fig. 12: The aiming point for your mallet

A summary of how to play a croquet stroke

(a) Decide where you want the croqueted ball to go, then draw an imaginary line back to where it is at the moment.

(b) Put your ball on this line, behind the other ball and touching it. The imaginary line should now pass through the centre of both balls (like line A in fig. 12).

(c) Decide where you want your ball to go.

(d) Aim halfway along a line (line D in fig. 12) joining the final positions of both balls.

(e) Strike your ball.

EXERCISES

1   Place two balls and your mallet in the same position as in fig. 12. Place two coins a few yards away on the two imaginary lines A and C. Judge the correct aiming point and strike your ball. Watch to see if the balls travel over the coins.

2   Repeat the exercise above for different angles.

You will have grasped the idea if you can regularly get the ball to cross within one foot of the coins.

Note: Do not make the angle too wide. Also, apart from noting where the balls come to rest so that you can judge line D, do not worry about the relative distances each ball travels. This is covered next.

Strength

Now you know how to get the balls to move in the correct directions. The next thing to master is getting them to travel the correct distances. To see why this is necessary, place two balls in contact for a croquet shot and then make the following experiments:

1   Strike your ball so that both move in the same direction. Note that your ball only goes about a quarter of the distance of the other.

2   Now strike at the angle shown in fig. 9. This time both balls travel approximately the same distance.

3   Finally, strike your ball at almost right angles to the other. The croqueted ball hardly moves while yours goes a long way.

The previous section of this chapter described how to calculate and play angled shots. In these experiments, the angle at which your ball moves in relation to the other varies from nothing, where both balls go in the same direction (experiment 1), through an angle (experiment 2) to almost 90 degrees – i.e. at right angles (experiment 3). It is *almost* 90 degrees, because at right angles or more, only your ball will move and the rules say that both balls must move. From this you can see that the nearer your angle is to 90 degrees the greater will be the movement of your ball in relation to the other.

So, although the relative distance that each ball will travel can be altered, to achieve this you have to alter the angle of shot as well. This is not a very satisfactory situation. You need to be able to control the relative distance that each ball travels independently of the angle. The way to do this is similar to snooker: you put varying amounts of spin on your ball when you strike it.

No spin

This is known as a *drive shot*. It is the normal shot described in Chapter 3 'Striking the Ball'. It should also have been the shot you used for the three previous experiments. No spin is put on your ball with this shot but that does not mean that it is no good. In fact there are many situations where it is exactly the right shot. Also, it is easier to play than the shots that do impart spin.

EXERCISES

1   Place two balls in contact and try some drive shots, sending both balls in a straight line, and observe what happens to each ball.

2   Try some drive shots at various angles and observe what happens to each ball.

Top spin

This is known as a *roll shot*. It puts top spin on your ball, making it go further than it otherwise would have done. To play a roll shot, slide your hands down the mallet shaft into the position demonstrated by Jill Waters in photograph 12 in the colour section. As mentioned in Chapter 3, putting your index finger down the mallet shaft is a matter of personal choice. Note that her finger does not actually touch the mallet head, because it would be a fault to do so. Now strike your ball and follow through in the manner illustrated in fig. 13, and photographs 13–14.

In photograph 13, Jill has taken stance and is ready to play the shot. Although a centre-style player, Jill plays roll shots from the side. This is because she, like many players, finds a centre-style roll shot too awkward. Note the position of her hands, feet and mallet, and also that her eyes are firmly fixed on her ball. To play the shot, Jill swings back, keeping her arms, hands and mallet together as a single unit, and her body still. Shen then swings forward, passing through the same position shown in photograph 13. As with other shots, follow-through is most important. Photograph 14 shows this. It also shows both balls travelling off together.

The amount of 'roll' that you obtain depends on a number of things.

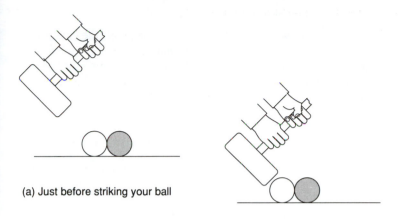

(a) Just before striking your ball

(b) At the point of striking your ball

Note: The position of the hands are shown for illustration only. For a more accurate view of hand positions, see the photographs which demonstrate the roll shot.

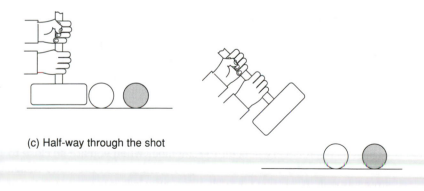

(c) Half-way through the shot

(d) The follow-through

Fig. 13: The roll shot

These are the two most important:

1   How far up your ball you hit it. Up to a certain point, the closer your mallet strikes to the top of the ball, the more the roll – i.e. the further your ball goes relative to the other. Beyond that point your ball digs into the ground and the shot is ineffective. Fig. 14 illustrates the range over which a roll shot works properly.

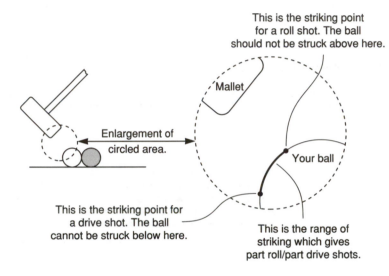

This is the striking point for a roll shot. The ball should not be struck above here.

Mallet

Enlargement of circled area.

Your ball

This is the striking point for a drive shot. The ball cannot be struck below here.

This is the range of striking which gives part roll/part drive shots.

Fig. 14: The effective range for a roll shot

2   How far down the shaft you hold the mallet. This is not precise but generally, the lower down you hold it, the more roll you can get. Remember that you are not allowed to touch or hold the mallet head.

The roll shot is not an easy one to master. To help you, here are some useful hints.

• Keep your eye on your ball. This has already been stressed in the last chapter, but it is very difficult to remember when you are so close to your ball and you are concentrating on getting all of the other things right as well. If you find yourself missing the ball or catching the top of it, you are probably moving your eye.

• Swing through smoothly. If you jerk at it the balls will squirt off in odd directions. If you stab into the ground, nothing much will happen!

- Swing through quickly. There can be a tendency to slow the swing down because you are so close to the balls. If you do this you will maintain contact with your ball for too long and push it in the direction of your mallet instead of it going off at the angle intended. As well as the shot going wrong it is also a fault to push your ball (this is true in all shots although it is most likely in the roll).

- Swing through in the right direction. Yet again, the closeness produces a tendency to swing in the direction you want your ball to go instead of the 'half-angle' point described earlier. You are probably making this fault if you find that your ball goes too wide in angled roll shots.

EXERCISES

1 Place two balls in contact and play a roll shot in a straight line so as to get both balls to travel five yards.

2 Try the same shot for ten yards.

3 Try some roll shots at various angles and observe what happens to each ball.

You will have grasped the idea if you can regularly:

- For 1: get both balls within one yard of where you want them.
- For 2: get both balls within three yards of where you want them.

Back spin

This is known as the *stop shot*. It has the opposite effect to a roll shot, i.e. your ball only travels a short distance compared to the croqueted ball. Snooker players can get back spin by striking under the cue ball. This is not possible in croquet as the mallet face is too big. Some small amount of spin can be achieved by dropping the mallet swiftly down to the ground at the exact point when your mallet strikes your ball.

Fig. 15 and photographs 15 and 16 illustrate the stop shot. Note in photograph 15 that although Celia is holding her mallet in the same way as for a drive or single-ball shot, the front of her mallet is raised very slightly. In photograph 16, Celia has just struck her ball. Note that her ball has moved only slightly, while the croqueted ball has moved a long way. Her mallet rests on the ground at the point of impact.

The amount of 'stop' that you get depends on two things:

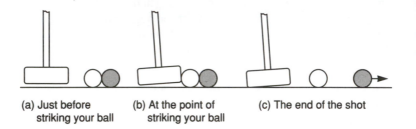

(a) Just before
    striking your ball

(b) At the point of
    striking your ball

(c) The end of the shot

Fig. 15: The stop shot

1 How quickly you stop the mallet after the mallet has struck your ball. The grounding of the mallet to give back spin helps achieve this but some people play stop shots by simply stopping the mallet in mid-swing just after it has struck the ball. In comparison tests that the author has carried out with a colleague there seems to be little difference in the results for either method. Choose therefore the method which you find easiest to play and gives the best results.

2 How quickly you drop your mallet. The quicker it is done the more the spin. However this is not a very important part of a stop shot so don't try too hard at it.

The stop shot may take some practice to master. To help you, here are some useful hints.

• Keep your eye on your ball. This is as true here as it is for the roll. If you don't, you will find your mallet stopping short of the ball.

• Keep the action smooth. The stop shot is of necessity one with a sudden finish but that does not mean it should be jerky. If you jerk at it the 'stop' action will not be as effective.

• It can often help with this shot if you move your feet a few inches back from your normal stance. Doing this helps you to lift the front face of your mallet as shown in fig. 15 and photograph 15.

EXERCISES

1 Place two balls in contact and play a stop shot in a straight line so as to make the croqueted ball travel ten feet while your ball travels one foot.

2 Try the same shot, making the distances ten yards and one yard.

You will have grasped the idea if you can regularly:

- For 1: get both balls within one yard of where you want them.
- For 2: get both balls within three yards of where you want them.

Side spin

Although a tiny amount of side spin can be put on your ball, it lasts for a very short time and has virtually no effect. For practical purposes side spin can be ignored.

A summary of the croquet stroke

Playing the complete croquet stroke can be summarised as follows:

D I R	(a) Decide where you want the croqueted ball to go, then draw an imaginary line back to where it is at the moment.
E C T	(b) Put your ball on this line, behind the other ball and touching it. The imaginary line should now pass through the centre of both balls (like line A in fig. 12).
I	(c) Decide where you want your ball to go.
O N	(d) Aim halfway along a line (line D in fig. 12) joining the final positions of both balls.
S T	(e) Note the distance that each ball has to travel.
R E N	(f) Remember that the wider the angle the more your ball will travel relative to the other.
G T H	(g) Decide how much 'roll' or 'stop' is needed.
	(h) Play the stroke.

The table opposite gives pointers to the type of shot to play by saying what happens in different situations.

Note: In Chapter 2, mention was made of the different characteristics of balls and mallets which were not of standard weight. If your set is like this, you will not get exactly the same results as those shown opposite. Play all of the shots and take careful note of any differences. Also see what type of stroke is needed so that the balls *do* move as described in the table.

EXERCISES

1 Play all of the shots in the table of distances on page 47. Do not worry too much about the strength of shot but check that the relative distances are as described in the table.

2 Play the shots again but this time choose appropriate distances for each ball, then try to play a shot with the correct strength to achieve your objective.

You will have grasped the idea if you can regularly:

* For 1: get both balls to do what the table says.
* For 2: get each ball to go where you want it plus or minus 30%.

Combination shots

As you start to improve at croquet strokes, try to combine some of them. By doing this you can get the two balls to move to exactly where you want them, instead of just somewhere nearby.

For example, suppose the angle you require is zero and that you want your ball to travel half the distance of the croqueted ball. The table opposite shows that when the angle is zero, a drive does not send your ball far enough if you get the croqueted ball right, while a roll sends it too far. You can combine a roll and a drive by sliding your hand only part way down the mallet shaft and by striking your ball half-way between the drive and the roll points (fig. 14). This shot is called a *half roll*. Other combinations give quarter roll, three-quarters roll, etc. If you look at photograph 13, Celia is playing a partial roll shot.

EXERCISES

1 Play the shot in photograph 13, varying the amount of roll until the shot produces the correct result shown in photograph 14.

Angle of shot (between balls)	What happens when you play:		
	A normal drive	A roll	A stop
Angle = 0° The balls are played in a straight line.	Your ball travels between a third and a quarter of the distance of the croqueted ball.	Both balls travel about the same distance.	Your ball travels about a tenth of the distance of the croqueted ball.
Angle = 10° The balls split apart a little.	Your ball travels about half the distance of the croqueted ball.	Your ball travels a bit further than the croqueted ball.	Your ball travels about an eighth of the distance of the croqueted ball.
Angle = 45° The balls split apart quite a lot.	Both balls travel about the same distance.	Your ball travels a lot further than the croqueted ball.	Your ball travels about half the distance of the croqueted ball.
Angle = 85° The balls split apart widely.	Your ball travels a long way while the croqueted ball hardly moves at all.	There is no point in playing a roll as a drive is better.	The stop has virtually no effect on your ball so play a drive shot.

Table of relative distances

2   Try a half roll sending the balls at an angle.

3   Choose three random points on the lawn. Take croquet from one of them
    and try to send the balls to the other two. See if you can find out what is
    possible and what is not.

Take-off shots

If you look at the table on page 47, you can see that when the angle is
large, the rules described so far break down. In fact what happens is that
your ball no longer splits off at an angle but goes in the direction in which
you strike it. It behaves almost as if there were no croqueted ball there.
This is actually rather useful! It means that if you want to leave the
croqueted ball where it is you can do so and just concentrate on your ball.

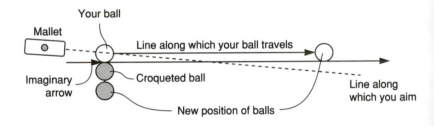

Fig. 16: The take-off shot

This type of shot is called the *take-off* because your ball takes off from the
other one, leaving it more or less where it was (but remember that for it
to be a legal shot, the croqueted ball must move – even if it is only a
fraction of an inch).

To play a take-off shot, refer to fig. 16. The balls are placed in contact
(this is still a croquet stroke), so that the imaginary arrowhead points in
the direction that you want your ball to go. Then, strike your ball in the
direction shown, imagining that you are striking just a single ball.

EXERCISES

1   Play a take-off shot, sending your ball ten yards while not moving the
    croqueted ball more than one foot.

2 From one corner spot, take-off to within five yards of another corner.

You will have grasped the idea if you can regularly:

* For 1: achieve the shot stated.
* For 2: achieve the shot stated without sending the croqueted ball off the court.

The continuation stroke

Having successfully played the croquet stroke, you now have one more stroke, the *continuation stroke*. This is used to do one of four things. The four options are given below in the order in which they are most likely to be chosen.

(a) To roquet another ball

You will then play a croquet shot.

However, you can only roquet a ball that you have not roqueted before. If you have already roqueted each of the other three balls without making a hoop, you cannot make any more roquets this turn. You must choose between options (b), (c), or (d).

(b) To run a hoop

Running a hoop not only gives you an extra shot, but also you are now allowed to make a roquet on each and any of the other three balls.

You will then play option (a), (b) or (c), but not (d), depending on the situation having run the hoop.

(c) To take position somewhere

You would do this if options (a) or (b) were not possible. Since your turn is going to end after this shot, the most likely place will be somewhere near your partner ball. This move is discussed in more detail in the next chapter.

You then have no more shots.

(d) To scatter another ball

This is the least likely shot to take. Nevertheless it is useful to note that even if you are not allowed to roquet another ball it is still permissible to knock it out of the way in much the same way as you can in golf croquet. The balls then remain where they lie (or are replaced if they go off court).

You then have no more shots.

EXERCISES

1   From various positions around a hoop, including behind it, do the following:

(i) Choose a direction in which to run the hoop.
(ii) Place two balls on your chosen spot, ready to take croquet. It is recommended that initially you do not play from closer than six inches or further than three yards from the hoop.
(iii) Play a croquet stroke so as to put your ball in front of the hoop ready to run it. The croqueted ball should be sent to the opposite side of the hoop and about two yards beyond it. An example is shown in fig. 17.

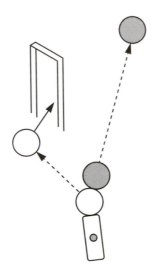

Fig. 17: Exercise 1

(iv) In your continuation shot, run the hoop.
(v) Having run the hoop, roquet the other ball again.

2   From various positions around the lawn, do the following:

(i) Place one ball (x) somewhere on the lawn.
(ii) Choose a spot from which to take croquet.
(iii) Place two balls on your chosen spot, ready to take croquet.

(iv) Decide where to send the croqueted ball.

(v) Play a croquet stroke so as to put your ball to within a yard of the previously placed ball (x). The croqueted ball should be sent to within a yard of its chosen spot. An example is shown in fig. 18.

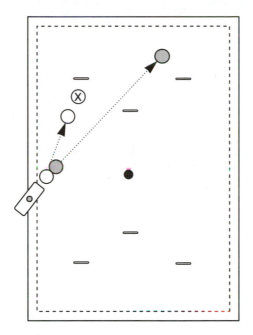

Fig. 18: Exercise 2

(v) In your continuation shot, roquet ball x.

You now know all of the basic strokes. It is time to start a game.

5

— MAKING A BREAK —

The first four chapters have given you an introduction to the game, how to choose and set out the equipment, the way to play shots, and detailed instruction on control of the balls. It is now time to consider an actual game. There are many ways to start a game but the one described here is used more than any other.

——————— Starting a game ———————

Fig. 19 shows the positions of the four balls when they have been put into play as described below.

The first ball on the lawn

You have chosen to start from the 'A' baulk. However, it is not a good idea to go straight for the first hoop. If you bounce off it you will leave an easy target for ball two. If you do make the hoop, what do you do next? You cannot safely shoot for hoop two as you will be close to the 'B' baulk if you miss. So you have to go somewhere safe. It is not worth the risk for just one hoop. The correct place to put ball one is near corner four. This makes a long shot for ball two. Even if hit, making hoop one from there is difficult.

The second ball on the lawn

Assume that ball one has been placed near corner four. For the reason described above, it is not very productive to shoot at ball one. Ball two should be placed to '*lay a tice*'. A tice, short for entice, is one which

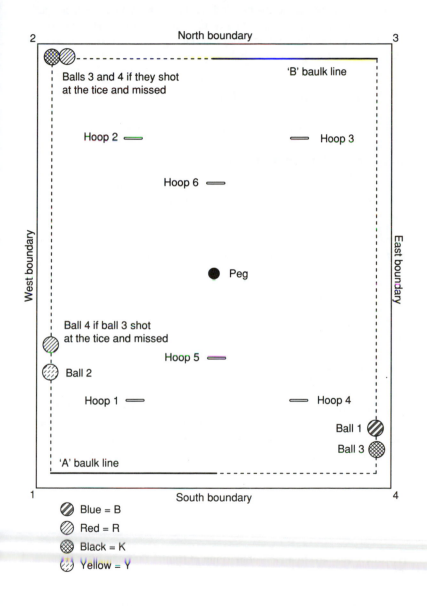

Fig. 19: Positions of the balls after the start of a game

tempts your opponent to shoot at it, but is sufficiently far away that he or she misses. Some cunning is needed here because you have to be a judge of what your opponent thinks is a tempting tice! A typical place to send your ball is along the west boundary about eight yards down from corner one. Shoot at this point from half-way along the 'A' baulk.

The third ball on the lawn

The player of ball three has two main choices now:

(a) Shoot at the tice from corner one

If this is hit, with your croquet stroke send ball two to about three-quarters of the way towards hoop two from hoop one. Then with your continuation stroke, 'join up' with ball one, i.e. put your ball close to it.

If, when you hit the tice, you happened to rush it to the correct position, play a take-off to ball one and roquet it with your continuation stroke. Then, in your next croquet stroke, roll both balls to a position about seven yards from corner four, down the east boundary. Finally, with your last continuation stroke, give yourself a foot-long rush to hoop one.

If you miss, you should have struck your ball sufficiently hard that it ends up in or near corner two.

(b) Join up with ball one

Shoot from the centre court end of 'A' baulk to put your ball off court so that it is replaced on the yard line about a yard away from ball one. By doing this you are putting the pressure on your opponent to hit his or her own tice (see below). Do not actually shoot at ball one: the chances of hitting are small and if you miss you could well leave a '*double target*'. A double target is two balls so close together they increase greatly the chance of the opponent hitting.

The fourth ball on the lawn

By now there are many combinations of things that can have happened. The two most common are:

(a) Ball three has shot at the tice and missed

Shoot at ball two from half-way along the 'A' baulk. If you miss, you are joined up. If you hit, roll to a *'guarded leave'* for hoop one. Guarded leaves are explained later in this chapter.

(b) Ball three has joined up with ball one

In this situation you cannot join up because doing so will leave two balls near hoop one which could be used by your opponent to make that hoop. So, as stated above, there is some pressure to hit the tice.

Shoot at your tice from corner one with sufficient strength to go to corner two if you miss. The reason for striking hard is that you do not want to have two balls close together near hoop one when your opponent is already joined up.

If you hit, play a take-off shot to balls one and three. Roquet one of them, then play a take-off shot to a position behind the other so that you have a rush to hoop one. With your continuation stroke roquet and rush to hoop one. (If this all seems a bit complicated, don't worry, the sequence is described in detail in the next section.)

In other words, by hitting the tice you have given yourself a chance of running hoop one and maybe hoop two and maybe . . . You are in fact starting a break.

—— The definition of a break ——

A definition of a break was given in Chapter 1:

With care and skill, it is possible to play so that the making of roquets, the subsequent croquet strokes, and the running of hoops all combine to produce a situation in which many hoops can be run in a single turn.

A turn where more than one stroke is played (and, hopefully, one or more hoops are scored) is called a break. It should be a player's objective at the start of a turn to make a break, because:

- by making a break, more hoops are likely to be scored.

- running several hoops in one turn gives your opponent less opportunity to score than running each hoop individually.

- scoring hoops in a break is often easier than scoring them individually.

- making a break is a very satisfying and rewarding thing to do. It also makes for a good game of croquet.

How to make a break

In this next section, and some others which follow, some time will be spent describing the movement of balls around a lawn. To make it easier to follow the diagrams, the following conventions have been used.

1 It is assumed that one player will be using red or yellow. This player will be called ROY. The other player will be using blue or black and will be called BOB.

2 To make things easier to see, hoops and balls are drawn much larger than they should be with regard to the scale of the lawn.

3 A key identifies the coloured balls on each diagram.

4 The initial and subsequent positions of balls are marked in curly brackets. The initial position on the diagram is always 1. So the initial position for red is shown as {R1}, etc. Black is shown as K {K1} to distinguish it from blue {B1}. Only significant movements are recorded on the diagrams to avoid cluttering them, so {R3} is the third significant position of red and not necessarily the third actual position in play. To help you understand what is happening, where there is a text description to go with a diagram, the significant positions are cross-referenced into the text.

The section above, 'Starting a game', finished with the player of ball four shooting at the tice. Assume that ROY is playing red and has hit this tice (yellow) {Y1}. This is shown opposite in fig. 20. BOB is close together near corner four {B1}{K1}. Yellow was originally in position {Y1} but was rushed to position {Y2} when red hit it. ROY takes off to BOB's balls near corner four. Because this shot is a take-off, yellow only moves a little, so this is not shown in the diagram. Red is struck from position {R1} (in contact with yellow) to position {R2}. From here he has an easy shot to roquet black. Black is rushed off court by this. It is replaced on the yard line {K2} and red prepares to take croquet from black.

A brief word on replacing balls on the yard line. Since the yard line is not marked on the lawn, it is a good idea to measure your mallet and note or mark on it a point which is one yard long. This will make replacement of the ball easier. Note that it is the centre of the ball which is placed on the yard line, not the inside edge.

Fig. 21 over the page gives the new position of the balls. Red plays a short take-off shot into the yard line area so as to obtain a perfect rush

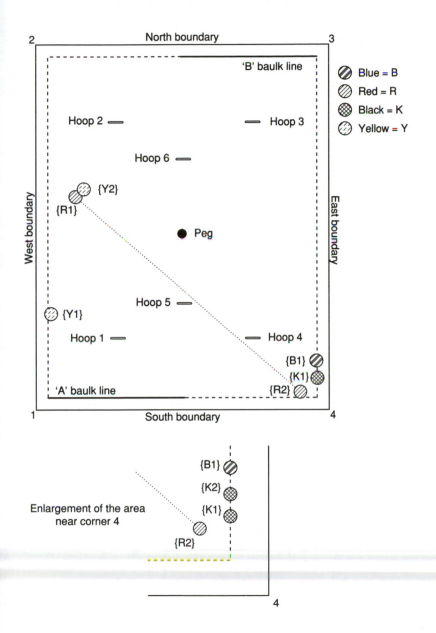

Fig. 20: Making a break after hitting the tice (a)

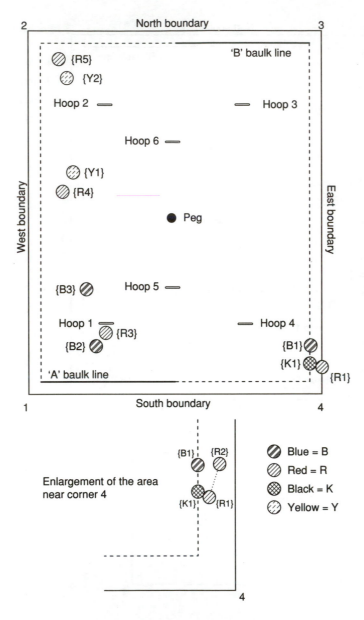

Fig. 21: Making a break after hitting the tice (b)

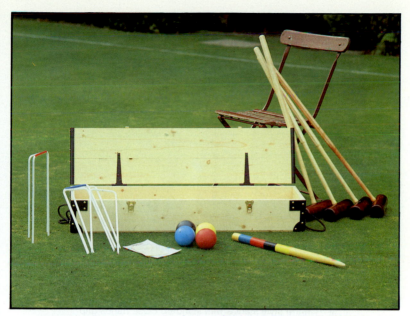

1 A croquet set

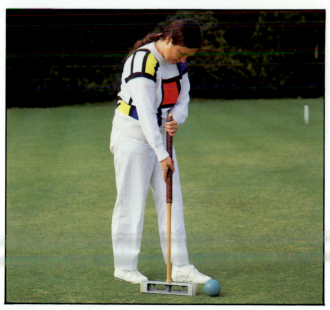

2 Side style stance with standard grip

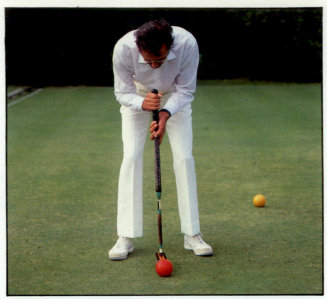

3 Centre style stance with standard close hands grip

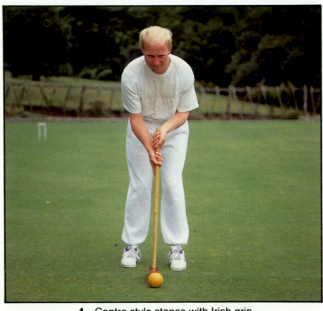

4 Centre style stance with Irish grip

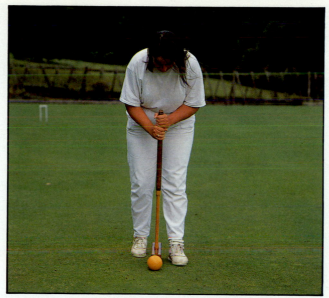

5 Centre style stance with Solomon grip

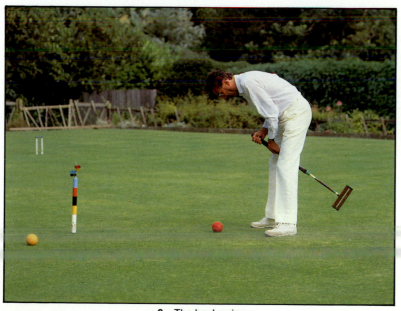

6 The backswing

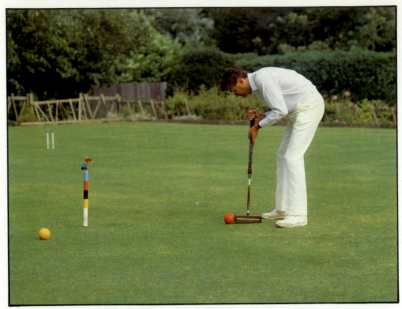

7 The strike

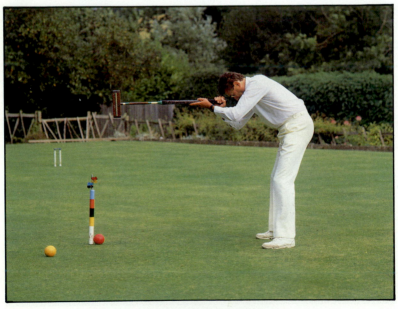

8 The follow-through

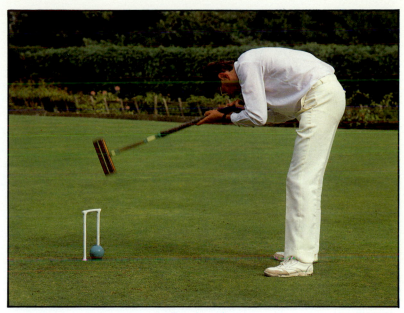

9　Running a hoop

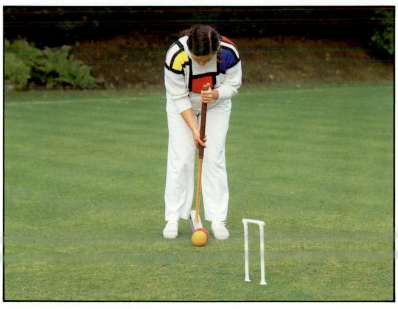

10　Croquet stroke approaching hoop

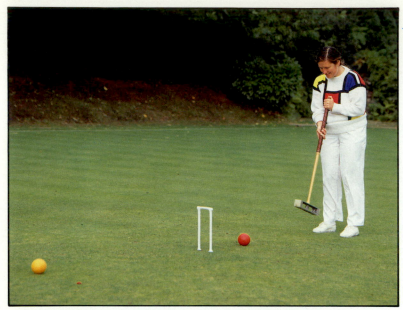

11 Croquet stroke final ball positions

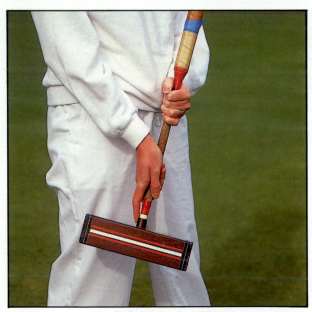

12 Roll shot hand positions

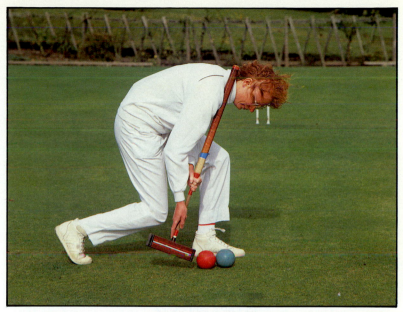

13　Roll shot stance

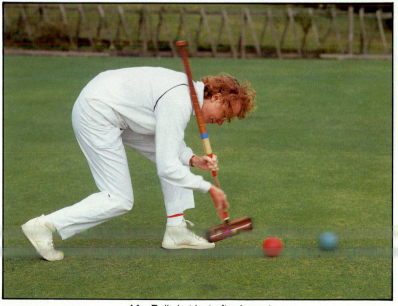

14　Roll shot just after impact

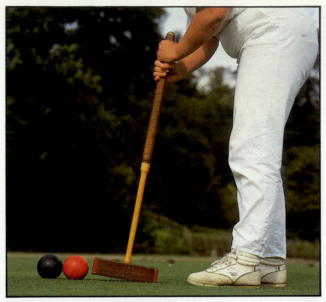

15 Stop shot stance

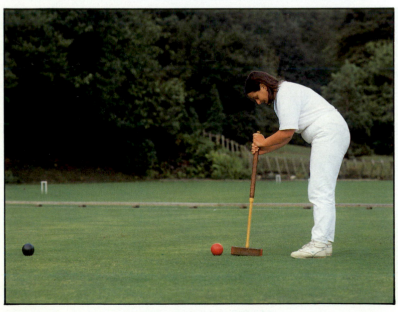

16 Stop shot at point of impact

towards hoop one, position {R2}. Note that red is *not* replaced on the yard line. The rule is explained in the boxed section.

The yard line rule

The yard line area is that part of the court which is between the yard line and the edge of the court, i.e. it is a one-yard strip round the inside edge of the court. Any ball which goes into the yard line area is replaced on the yard line at its nearest point to the ball when it has stopped moving (see fig. 3).

This rule does *not* apply to your ball when it is entitled to a continuation stroke. It is entitled to a continuation stroke after a croquet stroke and after running a hoop. In both of these cases if your ball goes into the yard line area it is played from where it lies.

So if you play a croquet stroke which sends both balls into the yard line area, the croqueted ball is replaced on the yard line but yours is not. (Note that if either ball goes off court, rather than in the yard line area, your turn ends. See Chapter 1, 'other rules'.)

So with your continuation shot you have a rush to hoop one {B2}. This is similar to the exercise on page 50 in Chapter 4, on roquets and rushes. If you achieve this, your objective will be to send blue beyond hoop one to position {B3}, while putting red in front of hoop one, position {R3}. This is similar to the exercise on page 51 in Chapter 4.

Red will now run hoop one. Blue has conveniently been placed on the far side of the hoop and is waiting to be roqueted (remember that having run a hoop, you can roquet all of the balls again). Red can then take-off for yellow near hoop two {R4}. With skill and luck, you will get a rush to hoop two and run it. If you do not, you can use the last croquet and continuation shots to set up a rush for red towards hoop two using yellow {R5}{Y2}.

So, the result of this turn has been the running of hoop one and possibly of hoop two. Not only that, you have separated blue and black and you have left an opponent's ball near yellow's hoop while having a rush to the red's next hoop. Not a bad start! You have made a break and retained control of the game.

EXERCISE

Set up balls in the positions shown in fig. 20, just after the tice has been hit. Follow the book and try to run hoops one and two. In this, and all exercises in this chapter, try to get each shot exactly as shown in the book. If it does not work, replace the balls for that shot and try again. Make three attempts at getting it right. If you still have not succeeded, place the balls in their correct positions and carry on, noting that this particular shot is one you should practise.

Problem 1

How might the above break be modified so that hoop three could be run in the same break? Play your solution and see if it works.

In this and other problems, it will help if you draw a diagram. If your solution is different to the one given in the book, try both – you could well come up with a better one! All problems assume a full-size lawn. If you have a smaller lawn, modify any distances given in the problems accordingly. Answers to this and all problems at the end of the chapter.

How to use the rush to create breaks

The rush is very useful when trying to make a break because if you have a good rush, you can send the roqueted ball where you want it. There have been a couple of examples of this already. In the first, where the tice was hit, red obtained a rush on blue that put blue in front of hoop one instead of near corner four. The second example formed part of the solution to Problem 1.

Another useful thing that you can do with a rush is to get behind a boundary ball, as in fig. 22 opposite. Suppose red is part-way along the east boundary, on the yard line and near hoop four {R1}. You have just run hoop two {B1}. You hoped to get a rush on yellow {Y1} (the ball you used to approach hoop two) towards hoop three. Unfortunately you did not, but you did get a rush towards red. A hard rush sends yellow off court near red. Yellow is replaced on the yard line {Y2} (remember, it is not a fault to rush the roqueted ball off court). A little take-off shot will now give you the required rush towards hoop three {B2,B3}.

The rush can also be used to give yourself easier croquet shots – see the next section under 'drive shots'.

So whenever you play a croquet stroke with the intention of moving your ball to a position where it can make a further roquet, look to see if a rush will help. If you already have a rush lined up, make sure that you know how hard you want it to be. Finally, if chance gives you a rush, don't just take it because it is there! Check first to see if you need one.

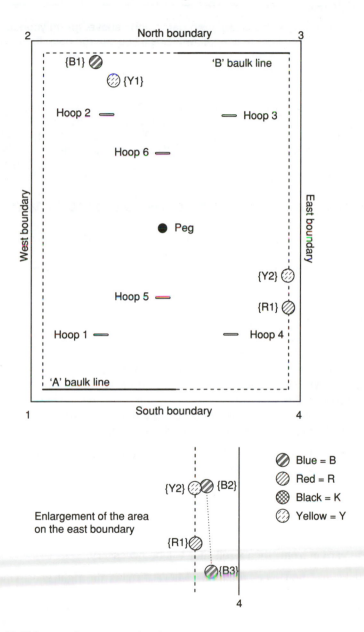

Fig. 22: Using a rush to create a break

EXERCISE

Place the balls as described three paragraphs above, giving yourself the rush towards red from near hoop two. See if you can run hoop three using red.

Problem 2

You are ROY and it is the start of your turn. Red has a perfect rush towards hoop four (its hoop) from near corner one. Black is in corner two, blue is one yard in front of hoop four. What do you do? The hoops required by the other balls may be assumed to have no significance in this problem.

How to use croquet strokes to create breaks

The rush is useful in creating breaks, but the croquet stroke is essential. To show how important the croquet stroke is, each type of shot is considered and examples of its use given. Refer back to Chapter 4 if necessary.

The drive shot

This is the shot that you should use whenever possible because it is the easiest to play and the most predictable. Use it when you are approaching your hoop from about a yard in front. By doing so you will send your ball the two feet needed to get a foot in front of your hoop, whilst the croqueted ball is sent forward about eight feet. When you have run your hoop, the other ball is waiting to be roqueted again. Not only that, you may well have a good rush to somewhere helpful.

Be on the look-out for rushes that give you useful break-making drive shots. An example can be found in the solution to Problem 1.

The roll shot

The need to play a roll shot often indicates a previous poor shot. If you fail to get a good rush to your hoop and end up five yards to the side instead of one yard in front, then a roll shot will be necessary.

There are, however, situations where a roll is the right shot. One of these is where you have made a roquet a long way from your hoop. You do not consider it worth while attempting the hoop, so you roll both balls to positions near the hoop and leave yourself a good rush for your next turn.

Another time when a roll is useful is if you are taking croquet from your ball in the middle of the lawn and wish to retire to a boundary with both of them.

You would also play a roll shot approach to a hoop that you were correctly in front of if you happened to want a rush backwards after running your hoop – perhaps to get to your ball on the boundary behind you. An example of this type of approach will be seen in Chapter 6 under two-ball breaks.

You can see from the above that the roll shot is used more often for recovery or safety than for break-building. Having said that, there are lots of times when recovery or safety shots are required, so practise your rolls!

The stop shot

Play a stop shot if your rush was too good and you are taking croquet from one foot in front of your hoop instead of one yard. That way you will still be able to get the croqueted ball a reasonable distance past your hoop.

A stop shot is also a good ploy if you wish to send the croqueted ball to a useful position, while keeping your ball near another one.

The take-off shot

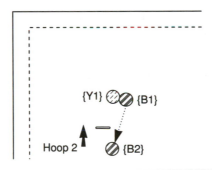

Fig. 23: Approaching a hoop from behind

Use a take-off shot to get in front of your hoop if you have rushed the roqueted ball the wrong side of your hoop, as in fig. 23. By doing this you will still have a ball waiting for you when you have run the hoop. You will not have much say in the position of the croqueted ball as a take-off leaves it almost where it lies. That is the penalty for not getting the rush right!

A take-off shot should also be used when you *want* the croqueted ball to remain where it is. For example: you are trying for hoop two. There is another ball already at hoop two. You are taking croquet from a ball at hoop three. You will want to leave the ball at hoop three where it is so that you can use it after running hoop two. So you play a take-off.

Play a take-off when you cannot send the croqueted ball anywhere useful. Such a situation might be if you were taking croquet from corner three and wished to reach a ball waiting at your hoop two. Any attempt at a roll over that distance is almost certainly doomed.

Opportunities for creating a break

Look out for:

- An opponent's balls left conveniently near your hoop. Try to avoid doing the same thing yourself!

- Opportunities to get a rush on one ball by taking off from another.

- Opportunities to create two-, three- and four-ball breaks. A two-ball break is created simply by getting a rush to your hoop. A three- or four-ball break is created by spotting croquet shots which set up the conditions described in the next sections. The solutions to both Problems 1 and 2 create three-ball breaks.

EXERCISE _____

Problem 3

Begin with the same situation as in Problem 2 except that the black ball is now one yard due east of hoop one. How would you achieve the following: yellow in front of hoop five, black near the peg, blue as yet untouched and red in a position to roquet blue?

_____

The two-ball break

This is a break using your ball plus one other. The other ball may be your own or the opponent's. It is the easiest break to set up because all you need is a rush to each hoop, but it is the hardest to maintain because of the accuracy required.

Fig. 24 shows a two-ball break from hoop three to hoop five, starting with

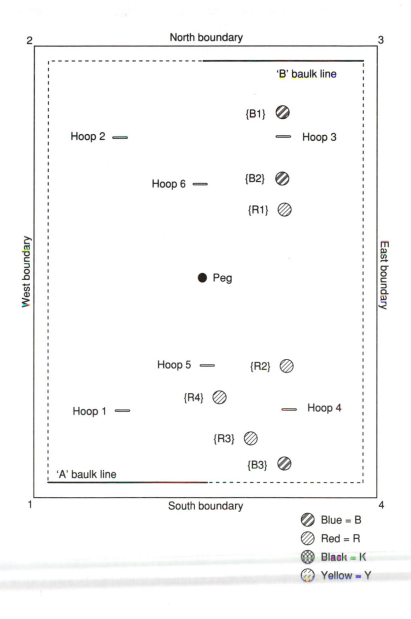

Fig. 24: A two-ball break

your ball in front of hoop three and the other ball beyond it. The letters and figures in curly brackets refer to those on the diagram. Only the key ball positions have been shown, to keep the diagram clearer. Your ball is blue {B1}, the other is red {R1}.

Here is the shot sequence:

1 Run hoop three getting a rush towards hoop four {B2}.

2 Rush red in front of hoop four {R2}.

3 Take croquet. In the croquet stroke put red beyond hoop four and a little to the right {R3}, while putting blue in front of hoop four.

4 Run hoop four getting a rush to hoop five {B3}.

5 Rush red to hoop five {R4}.

6 Take croquet. In the croquet stroke put red beyond hoop five . . .

The general principle of a two-ball break is to run your hoop and get a rush to the next one.

The sequence is quite easy to follow, but is very hard to execute. This is because the two-ball break relies on very accurate rushing, very good croquet stroke placing and very good control when running hoops.

EXERCISE

Set up the balls in the initial positions shown in fig. 24. Follow the sequence and try to run hoops three, four and five. As before, try to get each shot exactly as shown in the book. Make three attempts and if you still have not succeeded, carry on, noting that particular shot for practice.

Problem 4

How might this break be modified if yellow was on the south boundary, directly behind hoop four?

The three-ball break

This is a break using your ball plus two others, which may be your own or the opponent's. Fig. 25 (opposite) shows a three-ball break from hoop three to hoop five, starting with your ball in front of hoop three, one ball beyond hoop three and one ball in front of hoop four. Your ball is blue {B1}, red is as before {R1} and yellow is in front of hoop four {Y1}.

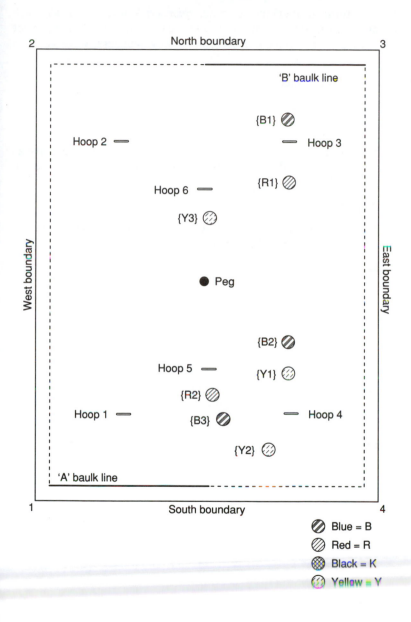

Fig. 25: A three-ball break

One new term occurs in the sequence: *pioneer*. A pioneer is a ball which is sent to your next hoop but one, ready and waiting for you when you get there. In the break you continually create new pioneers, while going to old or previous ones.

Here is the shot sequence:

1   Run hoop three.

2   Roquet red.

3   Take croquet. In the croquet stroke, send red in front of hoop five as a new pioneer {R2}, while putting blue close to yellow, the old pioneer {B2}.

4   Roquet yellow, rushing it to perfect position if necessary.

5   Take croquet. In the croquet stroke put yellow beyond hoop four {Y2}, while putting blue in front of hoop four.

6   Run hoop four.

7   Roquet yellow.

8   Take croquet. In the croquet stroke, send yellow in front of hoop six as a new pioneer {Y3}, while putting blue close to red, the old pioneer {B3}.

9   Roquet red . . .

The general principle of a three-ball break is to run your hoop, roquet a ball, then play a croquet stroke creating a new pioneer while getting in position to roquet the old one.

EXERCISE

Set up the balls in the initial positions shown in fig. 25. Follow the sequence and try to run hoops three, four and five.

Problem 5

What could you try that would make the break easier without adding to the risk of a breakdown? The answer does not involve the use of the fourth ball.

The four-ball break

This is a break using your ball plus all the others. It is the hardest break to set up because all of the balls have to be placed in the correct positions, but the simplest to maintain because once the balls are in position the shots are much easier.

Fig. 26 on page 70 shows a four-ball break from hoop three to hoop five, starting with your ball in front of hoop three, one ball beyond hoop three, one ball in front of hoop four and one ball by the peg. Your ball is blue {B1}, red and yellow are as before {R1}{Y1}, while black is near the peg {K1}.

One new term occurs in the sequence: *pivot*. A pivot is a ball which stays near the peg during a four-ball break.

Here is the shot sequence:

1 Run hoop three.

2 Roquet red.

3 Take croquet. In the croquet stroke, send red in front of hoop five as a new pioneer {R2}, while putting blue close to black, the pivot {B2}.

4 Roquet black.

5 Take croquet. Take-off to yellow, the old pioneer {B3}.

6 Roquet yellow, rushing it to perfect position if necessary.

7 Take croquet. In the croquet stroke put yellow beyond hoop four {Y2}, while putting blue in front of hoop four.

8 Run hoop four.

9 Roquet yellow.

10 Take croquet. In the croquet stroke, send yellow in front of hoop six as a new pioneer {Y3}, while putting blue close to black, the pivot {B4}.

11 Roquet black.

12 Take croquet. Take-off to red, the old pioneer {B5}.

13 Roquet red . . .

A four-ball break is very similar to a three-ball break. Pioneers are created and used in exactly the same way. Your ball, however, uses the pivot ball as an intermediate stop on the way to the old pioneer. The advantage of this is that having run a hoop and made the subsequent roquet, you only have one ball which needs to be sent accurately. This is the new pioneer. Your ball only has to stop somewhere near the pivot.

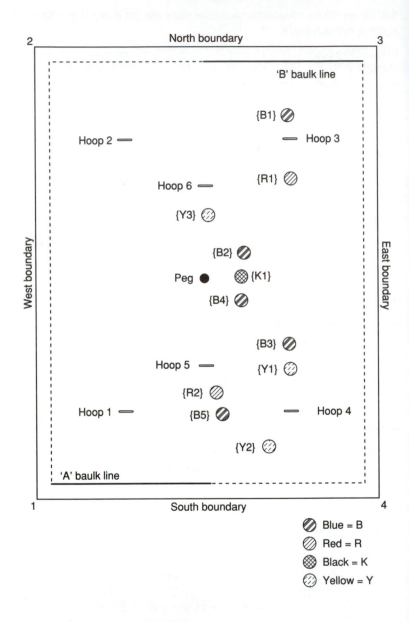

Fig. 26: A four-ball break

You then have a simple take-off shot from the pivot to get good position on the old pioneer.

EXERCISE

Set up the balls in the initial positions shown in fig. 26. Follow the sequence and try to run hoops three, four and five.

Problem 6

In the croquet stroke which was to have sent red in front of hoop five, you play a bad shot. Red only goes as far as the peg. Blue finishes one foot from black (the pivot) with a rush towards yellow. What could you do to restore the four-ball break?

The innings

When a player plays a turn in such a manner that control of the situation belongs to, and remains with, him or her, that player is said to 'have the innings'.

When you start your turn your aim is always to retain the innings if you have it, or to get the innings if you do not have it.

How to keep the innings

'End your turn with your balls united and those of your opponent separated.' This aspect of the game has given rise to many of the misconceptions about croquet, mentioned in Chapter 1. There are a few croquet players even today who believe that keeping one's opponent separated is the only important thing in the game. Hoop running comes a poor second to them and then only one at a time. Breaks are unheard of – much too dangerous! Sadly, new players are often beaten and disillusioned by these people because they do not have the experience to combat such play. If you should have this misfortune, shrug your shoulders and console yourself that few play like this.

So what is the difference between dull, negative play, and proper retention of the innings? Well, you can give your opponent long, difficult shots *and* be aggressive by putting one or both of his or her balls by your next or next-but-one hoops. It is not possible to be precise about this because much depends on the state of play – whose clip is where, etc.

You do not have to do this every time, indeed it may not be possible, but if you *are* separating your opponent, try to be constructive about it.

Do not leave double targets. This is very easy to forget if you are trying to end your turn with a rush for yourself. If you cannot get a rush without leaving a double target, consider leaving a rush for near where you think your opponent may join up. If you have left an aggressive leave as described above, make your rush point towards the ball that the opponent really does not want to move. Now he/she will either have to move it or else put the other ball in a corner. Either way, you keep control.

Make *guarded leaves*. A guarded leave is one where your balls are positioned in such a way that if your opponent shoots and misses, you can roquet the ball that has just missed and make a three-ball break from it. The classic guarded leave points are those which are about three yards diagonally inside the court from each corner towards the hoop that you wish to run. So, say you are trying for hoop two. The guarded leave point is three yards in from corner two. Your opponent shoots and misses. Roquet this ball and in the croquet stroke send it to hoop three, getting a rush on your other ball (which is waiting by hoop two) and thereby making a three-ball break. A guarded leave can be seen in fig. 21 {R5}{Y2}.

EXERCISE

Set up the balls in the guarded leave position described above and obtain a three-ball break by using a ball which is assumed to have just shot and missed. There is no need to run any hoops, just get a break set up. Try the same for the other corners.

Problem 7

Where is the guarded leave point for hoop five?

How to get the innings

The main thing to remember if you do not have the innings is – be patient. It is all too easy to panic when you have not taken croquet for about six turns and your opponent has made four hoops. You then make wild shots and give the game away. The game is not over until one person has pegged out both balls. I have seen a championship match in which one player had made all hoops and pegged out one ball, missing with the other, while his opponent had not scored a single hoop. The opponent then made a roquet and played two all-the-way-round three-ball breaks, to win the game.

The types of shot to play and whether to shoot or not are discussed in detail in the next section.

What to look for when you walk on court

When it is your turn to play, you must have a clear idea about which are the right sort of things to do and which are not. Sometimes the choice is quite easy. Your opponent breaking down at your hoop, leaving you an easy roquet is one example of an easy choice. Sometimes the choice is more difficult – should you take a shot that will give you an easy break if you are successful, but which will give your opponent an equally easy break if you fail? This section gives you some guidelines. Remember, though, the possible combinations of play are endless and what might be the right thing to do for one situation is wrong for another. This is as it should be. If the game became predictable it would be boring.

You should have been watching your opponent carefully. Therefore, when you walk on court, you know the state of play exactly. If for some reason you do not, find out what it is before doing anything. You can normally see the situation clearly by looking at the position of the clips and balls. If there is still any query, ask your opponent. You cannot of course ask your opponent what he or she intends to do next turn!

You will remember from Chapter 4 that there are four choices available to you when you have a continuation stroke after a croquet stroke or after running a hoop. There are similar choices when you play the first stroke of a turn (though, of course, scattering another ball does not apply at the start of a turn because as soon as you hit another ball you have roqueted it).

(a) To roquet a ball

You will then play a croquet shot.

If you are joined up, or have been left a simple roquet on an opponent's ball, then this is an easy choice and you will definitely take this option.

Before you do so, consider the rush. Would a rush help you, and if so, how hard should the rush be? Would it be better not to play a hard rush and instead play a take-off somewhere? Is the apparently obvious ball to play with the right one? It is very easy to think 'Ah, I have a rush with black to black's hoop. Black is the ball to play', ignoring two balls conveniently placed to give an easy break of two hoops or more with blue. The solution to Problem 3 is an example of this.

If you are not joined up, things get more tricky. There is a very useful little question to ask yourself before taking any shot: 'If I am successful with this shot, what benefits will I gain from it? If I fail, what benefits will my opponent gain?'. This question applies particularly when attempting difficult roquets, but can often be asked in other situations. It may stop you from taking suicidal shots which gain you almost nothing if you make a roquet but which give your opponent a three hoop break, or more, if you miss.

If your opponent has left one of your balls near one of his or her hoops, you should move it. If both your balls have been left at an opponent's hoops, move the one which gives your opponent the easiest break.

If you are left with one ball on the boundary and one in the middle of the lawn, move the one in the middle of the lawn.

If joining up (see option (c)), even widely, looks as though it would make things too easy for your opponent, consider shooting at one of your opponent's balls. The best of this type of shot is what is known as a *free shot*. This is one where you shoot hard, so that if you miss your ball carries on to end up harmlessly on a boundary a long way away.

If you do not have a free shot, see if you have a double target. Such a target considerably increases the chance of making a roquet. However, it does not make it certain! A double target 20 yards away is not going to be hit much more often than a single ball.

If you do not have a free shot or a double target, you might have a *safe shot*. A safe shot is one where even if you miss and land near your opponent, the opponent cannot do much with the situation.

(b) To run a hoop

As you will recall from Chapter 4, this is not very common at the start of a turn but it can happen. Running a hoop gives you an extra shot.

You will then play option (a), (b) or (c), depending on the situation having run the hoop.

If you have been left smack in front of your hoop, then usually you run it. Don't however take on a very difficult shot, particularly if the hoop in question is also your opponent's, or one of your opponent's balls is nearby. Also, if your other ball is within easy roqueting distance of your opponent, running the hoop and then not having an easy roquet yourself is a bad idea.

(c) To take position somewhere

If either making a roquet or running a hoop are not possible, or to attempt them would be too dangerous, either join up or go somewhere safe.

You then have no more shots.

If your opponent is joined up and you are not, do not join up too closely yourself. If you do, you give your opponent an easy pair of balls with which to get a rush (like the tice hit at the beginning of this chapter). Instead, give yourself a *wide join*. To create a wide join position your ball so that it is at a distance from which you would expect to hit most, but not all, of the time. Five yards is a typical figure, but this of course varies with individual ability.

Finally, if none of the above seems like a good idea, then look for the safest corner or boundary and retire to it. The safest place is where you are a long way from your opponent and his or her hoops. Occasionally there just isn't anywhere safe. Then you have to be bold, go for the best shot available and hope that you hit it!

EXERCISE ───────────────────────────────

Problem 8

As befits the final problem, this is a big one!

Set up the balls and clips as follows (fig. 27 on page 76). Yellow is one yard north-east of hoop two, with its clip on hoop one. Red is three feet from yellow with a rush to hoop two, and its clip on hoop two. Blue is halfway between hoops three and four, its clip on hoop two. Black is one yard in from the 'A' baulk (two yards in from the boundary), slightly to one side of hoop one, with its clip on hoop one. Blue and yellow are hidden by hoop six. Black and yellow are hidden by hoop two. All other balls are clear.

1 If it is ROY's turn, what are the options? For each option, answer the

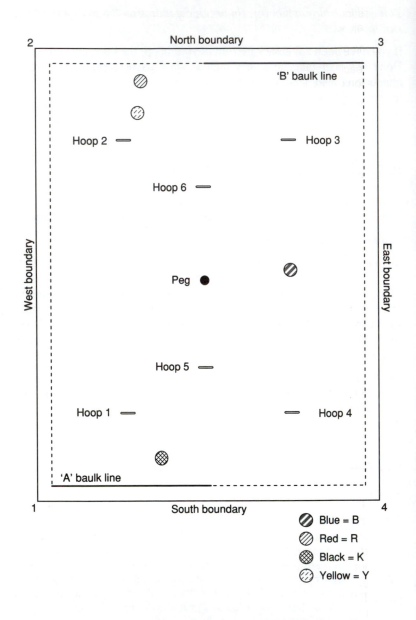

Fig. 27: Problem 8

question 'If I am successful with this shot, what benefits will I gain from it? If I fail, what benefits will my opponent gain?'.

2 Same problem, but now assume that it is BOB's turn.

Try out each situation, giving yourself success first, then failure. See if your estimation of the benefits/losses are justified.

All of the exercises given in this book have been designed to be played individually if you want (or have) to, although it is often helpful to have others around. This final exercise can also be played individually if no-one is available, but it is much better played in twos because you then have to start thinking about an opponent's ability to play as well as your own. If you do play in pairs, pretend to be BOB or ROY alternately to get more practice.

Conclusion

This has been a long chapter and many new ideas have been presented. Don't worry if you didn't understand everything the first time through. You are certainly not expected to be able to do everything. This will take time and a fair amount of practice. When you do have a good understanding, you will be well on your way to becoming a competent croquet player.

You should now be in a position to play a complete game of croquet except for the finish. That is the subject of the next chapter.

Solutions to problems

You will have noticed that in this chapter things are much less precise. There is talk of 'increase the chance' and 'safest place'. This is because each situation described depends on the strokes working correctly. Often they work partly. Often one ball goes the right way but the other does not. The solutions below also rely on everything happening as intended. If all the shots described go exactly as planned, the solution will work. If they do not, it still might work but will be more difficult. So do not think that these solutions are model answers that offer the perfect way to play. You may well see an equally effective solution, even a better one. Well done if you do!

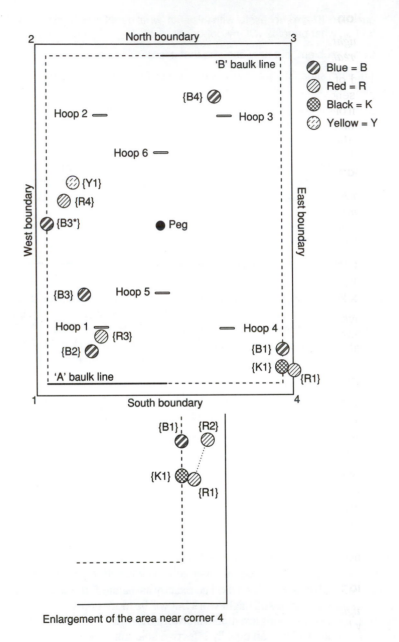

Fig. 28: Solution 1 – continuing the break after hoop two

Solution 1 (fig. 28)

How might the above break be modified so that hoop three could be run in the same break?

Instead of taking off from blue {B3} to yellow, play a croquet stroke which sends the blue to hoop three {B4} and puts your ball to a rush position on yellow {R4}. Things would be even better if you had obtained a rush on blue at {B3} to near the west boundary {B3*}. Your croquet shot is then a straight drive rather than an angled part-roll.

Solution 2

You are ROY and it is the start of your turn. Red has a perfect rush towards hoop four (its hoop) from near corner one. Black is in corner two, blue is one yard in front of hoop four. What do you do? The position of all other clips may be assumed to have no bearing on this problem.

Do not take the rush to hoop four. Instead, rush yellow to the east boundary beyond hoop four. In the croquet stroke, play a half roll, sending yellow to hoop five and red to blue.

You have now put the balls in positions which are described as a three-ball break. The three-ball break is very useful and is described in detail on page 66.

Solution 3 (fig. 29)

Begin with the same situation as in Problem 2 except that the black ball is now one yard due east of hoop one. How would you achieve the following: yellow in front of hoop five, black near the peg, blue as yet untouched and red in a position to roquet blue?

Rush yellow a couple of yards {Y2}. In the croquet stroke, send yellow to hoop five {Y3}, getting a rush to the peg on black {R2}. Rush black to near the peg {K2}. In the croquet stroke, take-off to blue {R3}.

You have now put the balls in positions which are described as a four-ball break. The four-ball break is the most useful break you can have and is described in detail on page 68.

Solution 4 (fig. 30)

How might the above break be modified if yellow was on the south boundary, directly behind hoop four?

When approaching hoop four, play your croquet stroke so that red is sent

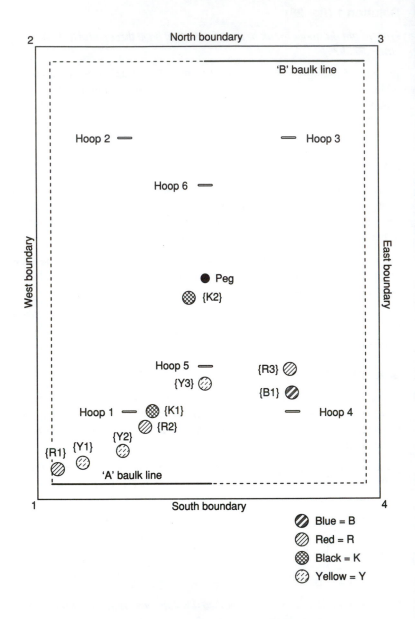

Fig. 29: Solution 3 – positioning balls for a break

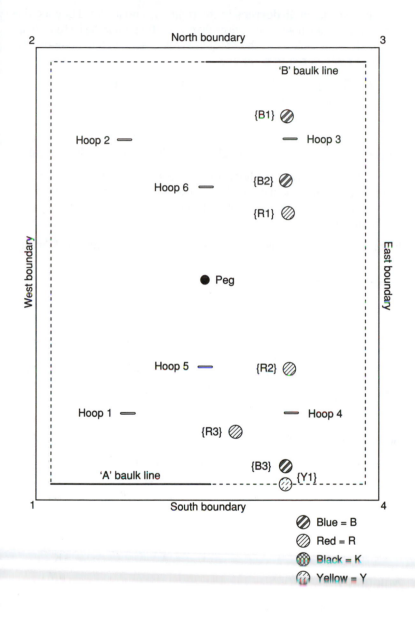

Fig. 30: Solution 4 – a modified two-ball break

at an angle of about 45 degrees to the right and about a yard beyond the hoop {R3}. Run hoop four fairly firmly so that your ball stops near yellow. Roquet yellow. In the croquet stroke, send yellow to hoop six, getting a rush on red to hoop five.

Note 1: When you run hoop four, if your ball continues off court, it is replaced on the yard line and you continue your turn.

Note 2: If your ball does not go off court but stops in the yard line area, your continuation shot is played from where it lies – it is not replaced on the yard line (see earlier in this chapter under 'How to make a break').

Note 3: If your ball runs the hoop and roquets yellow in the same stroke, you take croquet immediately. This is true whenever you run a hoop and make a roquet in the same stroke. The continuation stroke for running the hoop is lost.

If you succeed in the rush, you have created another three-ball break.

Solution 5 (fig. 31)

What could you try that would make the break easier without adding to the risk of a breakdown? The answer does not involve the use of the fourth ball.

The answer to this problem was given as part of the answer to Problem 1. If you can obtain a rush on the other ball having run a hoop, you will be able to play much easier croquet strokes. In the diagram, which is a partial repeat of fig. 25, the rush on red to a point near yellow {R1*} gives a much better shot than from its original position {R1}.

Solution 6

In the croquet stroke which was to have sent red in front of hoop five, you play a bad shot. Red only goes as far as the peg. Blue finishes one foot from black (the pivot) with a rush towards yellow. What could you do to restore the four-ball break?

Rush black to a few yards past yellow. In the croquet stroke, send black to hoop five and blue near yellow.

Solution 7

Where is the guarded leave point for hoop five?

Three yards from the south boundary, in front of hoop five. This solution is only true if your opponent's balls are somewhere separated towards

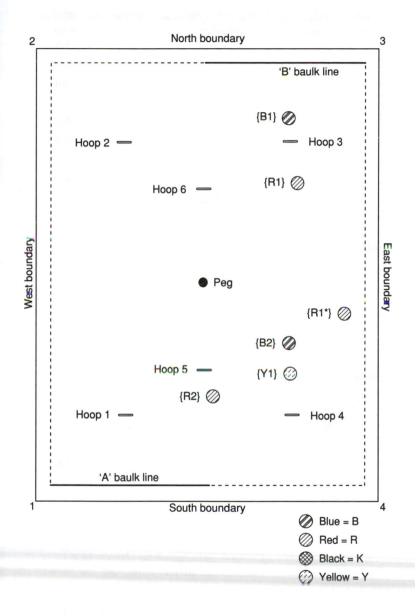

Fig. 31: Solution 5 – an improved three-ball break

the north boundary. If they are not then near corner one or four, as appropriate, gives a partially guarded leave.

Solution 8

1 *If it were ROY's turn, what are the options? In each case, how do the questions 'If I am successful with this shot, what benefits will I gain from it? If I fail, what benefits will my opponent gain?' get answered?*

Red playing

(a) Going safe or shooting at anything other than yellow is daft, so these choices can be ignored.

(b) Shooting at yellow gives a very good chance of making hoop two and a very good chance of a safe leave, even a guarded leave afterwards. There is little the opponent can gain from this specific shot. This is a good safe choice.

Yellow playing

(a) Going safe or shooting at anything other than red is as daft as it was for red at yellow, so these choices can be ignored.

(b) Shooting at red gives a possible chance of making hoop one off black by playing take-offs to blue, then black. Red is left near hoop two, giving the potential for a four-ball break since blue is near the middle. However, black is only two yards in from the boundary and it is a long journey from red. The benefits are great if you succeed but potentially dangerous if you fail (depending of course on how you fail). This is an adventurous and slightly hazardous choice.

2 *If it were BOB's turn, what are the options? In each case, how do the questions 'If I am successful with this shot, what benefits will I gain from it? If I fail, what benefits will my opponent gain?' get answered?*

Black playing

(a) Moving black seems reasonable if you think that choice (b) above would still be made by ROY, even if blue were moved. Going into corner four is very defensive, and gives no chance of a turn. It is however very safe. The benefit to you is nil, but the loss to the opponent is a potential three-ball break. This is a defensive choice.

(b) Shooting at blue gives a partially free shot, going off along the east boundary, yet giving the chance of a roquet. The benefit to you if you hit is a long shot at a break by taking off to red and yellow, using them to get a rush to hoop one. You have also separated your opponent. The benefit to the opponent if you miss is a possible break chance using red. This is a calculated risk choice.

(c) The yellow/red part double is 30 yards away and gives no better chance of a break if you hit and a moderate chance for your opponent to pick up a four-ball break if you miss. From black's point of view, ROY has a partially guarded leave. This shot gains little and could lose much. It is a bad choice.

(d) Trying to run hoop one is likely to result in you bouncing off the hoop, leaving ROY an easy three-ball break. It is a bad choice.

Blue playing

(a) Moving blue seems reasonable if you think that yellow choice (b) above would not be made by ROY. Going into corner four is very defensive, and gives no chance of a turn but it does provide a chance for black to join wide next time, and it is very safe. The benefit to you is little, the loss to the opponent little. This is a long-term defensive choice.

(b) Shooting at black puts two balls near hoop one if you miss, but a chance to take-off to two balls at your hoop if you hit. The benefit to you is a three-ball break chance. The benefit to your opponent is an excellent three-ball break chance. This is a reckless choice.

(c) Joining wide with black gives virtually the same chance of a three-ball break to ROY without even the long shot at a roquet that (b) gave you. This is a thoughtless and foolish choice.

(d) Shooting at red gives an excellent chance of a three-ball break if you hit and an equally excellent chance for your opponent to pick up a three-ball break if you miss. From blue's point of view, ROY has a guarded leave. This shot could gain much and could lose much. It is an aggressive and dangerous choice.

So there are the choices. Nothing is certain, no option is guaranteed. I know my own skills and would have my own preferred choice, but other players could well choose differently. Sometimes the choices are easy, sometimes very hard, but each time a ball is moved, the choices alter. Croquet is a fascinating game!

6

— FINISHING A GAME —

———— The rules for pegging out ————

It has already been noted in previous chapters that until a ball has run all of its hoops, it can neither be pegged out nor cause another ball to be pegged out. Although it would be perfectly legal for ROY to peg out yellow in one turn, and red in another, a better way is to wait until both balls have run all hoops. Then, by some means (discussed in a moment), ROY, here playing red, arranges for the final roquet to be made on yellow, rushing it near to the peg. With the croquet stroke, yellow is pegged out and removed from the court. Finally, with the continuation stroke, red is pegged out.

However, a few oddities can arise as follows:

- If ROY rushes yellow towards the peg (with the idea of finishing as described above) and yellow hits the peg, his turn immediately finishes. This is because a rushed ball can score a point against the peg just as it can when it is rushed through a hoop (a rush peel). Since the peg point has been scored, yellow has been pegged out. It is removed from the game and ROY has nothing from which to take croquet!

- If, in the croquet stroke in which yellow is pegged out, yellow bounces off the peg and moves red, or any other ball, nothing is replaced. Yellow is still removed and ROY's continuation shot played. If you spot that this is going to happen in your game, let it. Do not try to stop the collision, as it is a legitimate part of the game.

- If, in the croquet stroke, both balls hit the peg, both are pegged out and the game ends.

- It is perfectly legitimate to peg out any opponent's ball which has also run all of its hoops. This is a tactical move (see the section later on pegging out tactics). In the example above, ROY could peg out blue if it had run all of its hoops.

— Pegging out from a two-ball break —

In this and also in the three/four-ball break situations which follow, the break will start at hoop five, with your taking croquet in front of hoop five. Whether this is the start of your turn or whether you are in the middle of a longer break does not matter for the purpose of the discussion. It is also assumed throughout that your other ball has run all of its hoops and can therefore be pegged out.

You are ROY playing with red {R1} (see fig. 32 over the page).

(a) The other ball is yours {Y1}

In the croquet stroke, put yellow about three-quarters of the way to the peg {Y2} while putting red in front of hoop five. Run hoop five, getting a rush for hoop six on yellow {R2}. Rush yellow in front of hoop six {Y3}. Take croquet and in the croquet stroke, put yellow level with hoop six and to the side by a few inches {Y4}, while putting red in front of hoop six. Run hoop six by about three feet, getting a rush on yellow towards the peg {R3}. Rush yellow to near the peg {Y5} and peg out as described above.

(b) The other ball is an opponent's ball

Play hoop five as described above. For hoop six, in the croquet stroke, put blue in such a position that when you have run hoop six {R3}, you have a rush on blue {B4} to your *other* ball {Y1}. Take-off from blue to your other ball so that you have a rush towards the peg. Peg out as described above.

- Pegging out from a three-ball break -

(a) Your other ball is the one at hoop five

You are therefore taking croquet from yellow in front of hoop five {R1}{Y1} and blue is in front of hoop six {B1} (see fig. 33 on page 89). In the croquet stroke, put yellow about three-quarters of the way to the peg {Y2} while putting red in front of hoop five. Run hoop five, getting a rush

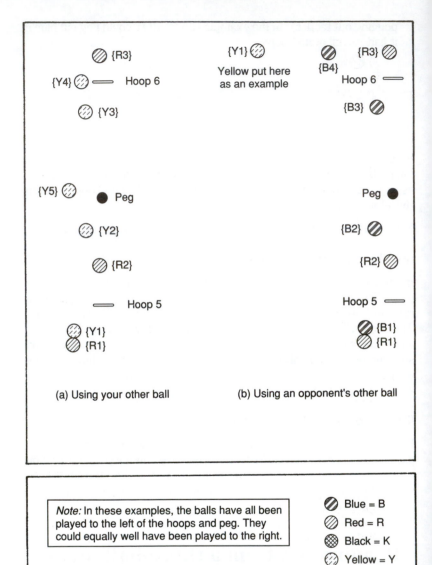

(a) Using your other ball

(b) Using an opponent's other ball

Note: In these examples, the balls have all been played to the left of the hoops and peg. They could equally well have been played to the right.

Blue = B
Red = R
Black = K
Yellow = Y

Fig. 32: Pegging out from a two-ball break

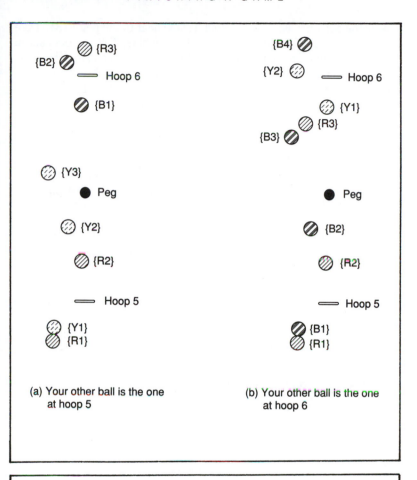

(a) Your other ball is the one at hoop 5

(b) Your other ball is the one at hoop 6

Note: In these examples, the balls have all been played to the left of the hoops and peg. They could equally well have been played to the right.

⊘ Blue = B
⊘ Red = R
⊗ Black = K
⊘ Yellow = Y

Fig. 33: Pegging out from a three-ball break

to near the peg on yellow {R2}. Rush yellow near to the peg {Y3}. Take croquet and take-off to blue at hoop six. Roquet blue. Take croquet and in the croquet stroke, put blue a few feet beyond hoop six and to the side by about a foot {B2}, while putting red in front of hoop six. Run hoop six by about a yard, getting a rush on blue towards yellow {R3}. This rush is not too critical. Take-off for yellow near the peg and peg out.

(b) Your other ball is the one at hoop six

You are therefore taking croquet from blue in front of hoop five {R1}{B1}, and yellow is in front of hoop six {Y1}. In the croquet stroke, put blue about three-quarters of the way to the peg {B2} while putting red in front of hoop five. Run hoop five, getting a rush to near yellow on blue {R2}. Rush blue near to yellow {B3}. Take croquet and in the croquet stroke send blue two yards beyond hoop six {B4} and red near yellow {R3}. Roquet yellow. Take croquet and in the croquet stroke, put yellow to the left of hoop six by about a foot and just beyond it {Y2}, while putting red in front of hoop six. Run hoop six and roquet blue. Take-off, getting a rush to near the peg with yellow and peg out.

– Pegging out from a four-ball break –

(a) Your other ball is not the one at hoop six

You are therefore either taking croquet from yellow in front of hoop five, or yellow is the pivot ball. Blue and black occupy the other positions of the break. In either case, continue the four-ball break, making sure that yellow is left near the peg. Run hoop six and take-off either directly or via the opponent's balls for yellow near the peg and peg out.

(b) Your other ball is the one at hoop six

You are therefore taking croquet from blue or black in front of hoop five and yellow is in front of hoop six. The method of play is the same as for the three-ball break (b) except that you have an extra ball to use.

EXERCISES

Set up each of the six situations described above and successfully peg out both balls.

You should be able to achieve a peg out about 50 per cent of the time.

The tactics of pegging out

Ideally, you will be able to complete the last hoops and peg out as described above and your opponent will get no more chances. When this does not happen and you are left with two clips on the peg, some strategy is called for.

(a) You have the innings

You should be attempting to leave your opponent widely separated, while you have a rush to the peg. The difficulty is to achieve this but not leave a double target. If you do leave a double target, your opponent will shoot; see (b) below.

If your opponent is separated and you don't have a rush to the peg, roll up close and peg your ball out. You then hope that your opponent misses so that you can peg the other ball out next turn!

(b) You do not have the innings

If both your opponent's balls are for the peg, then something needs to be done quickly. There is a very useful rule here.

If in your estimation your opponent is certain to finish next turn, try for the shortest roquet shot available to you. If your opponent may go out but it is not certain, join up.

However, if your opponent leaves you a double target, shoot for it anyway, unless your balls are quite close to each other.

(c) Pegging out an opponent's ball

Sometimes you will find that your opponent has got as far as the peg with one ball, while the other has some way to go. If you then reach the peg with one ball of your own, it can be useful to peg out the opponent's ball but not your own. The opponent then has nothing to join up with and must either shoot at you to make a hoop or try to get round without being able to roquet anything.

Tactics for the player of the two balls
Stay together, but do not leave any easy targets for the single ball. Do not use the opponent's ball unless an obvious three-ball break can be constructed or you have to move it out of the way. Remember that if you do not move the single ball, you can hide behind hoops without conceding a lift shot (described on page 108).

Tactics for the player of the single ball

Be aggressive. Shoot for your opponent every time unless to do so and miss is absolute suicide. If shooting is too dangerous, lurk on a boundary near your opponent's next hoop. If your opponent becomes separated or wired, take position in front of your hoop.

You are now in a position to play a complete game of croquet. The next chapter looks at how to put time limits on a game and how to even out different playing standards by handicapping.

7

SCORING AND HANDICAPS

—— Scoring and timing games ——

A game which is played to its conclusion no matter how long it takes will finish when one player (one pair in doubles) pegs out both balls. This means that the winner will have scored fourteen points – six hoops plus the peg for each ball. The loser will have scored less than this. The winner is therefore said to have won by fourteen points to X. X is the score of the loser.

Another way of expressing the result is to take X from fourteen and say that the winner has won by plus Y, where Y equals fourteen minus X.

Example
BOB pegs out both balls when ROY has clips on hoop four and peg. BOB has scored fourteen points, ROY has scored nine points. BOB has won by fourteen to nine (or BOB has won by plus five).

Timed games

Because untimed games can take a long time (the author knows personally of one game which took seven hours), players can agree on a time limit before starting. If there is a winner before time is up, the scoring is as above. If not, then each player (or side) adds up the total number of points and the one with the most points wins.

Example

After time ROY has clips on hoops two and six while BOB has clips on hoops one and three. ROY has scored six points, BOB has scored two points. ROY has won by six to two on time (or ROY has won by plus four on time).

The rules on the finish of a timed game are as follows:

1   Players agree on the clock or watch used for timing and the time at which to finish, before the game starts.

2   If there is no-one to watch the clock, the player not in play does the watching.

3   At the exact point when time is up, the watcher calls *'time'*.

4   The player in play when time is called is allowed to finish his or her turn. The opponent then also has one more turn. Unless there is a tied score, the game is over.

5   If there *is* a tie, the game continues until just one more point is scored by a player. That player then wins by plus one on time.

Example

When time is called ROY is in play with yellow and is about to run hoop four. The red clip is on hoop three. ROY runs hoop four with yellow but fails to run hoop five. BOB has one more turn. The black clip is on hoop four, the blue on hoop two. BOB hits in with blue and runs hoops two and three but fails to run hoop four. Both players have now scored six points. It is a tie. Play continues. ROY fails to hit in and BOB runs hoop four with blue.

BOB wins by seven points to six on time (or BOB wins by plus one on time).

A longer game

This book has described a game in which six hoops are run in a single direction by each ball, plus two peg points, giving a fourteen-point game. It is possible to make a longer game by running each hoop in both directions. This gives twelve hoops plus a peg point for each ball making a 26-point game. The route for this longer game is given in fig. 34 on page 104. This version is the one most often played at clubs.

The order of hoops is: hoops one to six as before, then:

one-back (hoop two in the reverse direction),
two-back (hoop one in the reverse direction),
three-back (hoop four in the reverse direction),
four-back (hoop three in the reverse direction),
five-back – called *penultimate* (hoop six in the reverse direction),
six-back – called *rover* (hoop five in the reverse direction),

and finally, the peg.

Readers should note that this longer or full game, as it is known, can take a long time to play, especially on a larger lawn. It is not recommended that you play a full game until you can regularly make breaks of three or four hoops.

Handicaps

It will not be very long, in a family or group of friends, before some players play better than others. This is so with any competitive game. To avoid the better players becoming bored and the less able players frustrated, a handicap system exists which balances abilities. This system allows the weaker player to have a certain number of extra turns, the amount varying according to the difference in ability.

Bisques

An extra turn is called a *bisque* turn and a player opting for such a turn is said to *take a bisque*. The section on page 97 explains how to work out the correct number of bisque turns to be played in any one game. To keep track of the number of bisque turns a player has left, small sticks, called bisques, are stuck into the ground at some convenient point at the edge of the lawn. Any odd sticks will do, paint them white and cut them into pieces about a foot long. Typically about 20 bisques will be enough for a single croquet set.

How to take a bisque

You can take a bisque immediately after the end of your ordinary turn. You must play with the ball that you have just been using – you cannot change to your other ball.

Example 1
You are playing with red. You are trying to run hoop three. Unfortunately

you stick in the hoop. Your turn ends, but you have a bisque. By taking your bisque you can start a new turn immediately and continue through the hoop.

Example 2
You shoot at your opponent on the boundary and just miss. Your ball is replaced on the yard line next to your opponent. Your turn ends, but you have a bisque. By taking your bisque you can start a new turn immediately and roquet your opponent.

The effect of taking a bisque

A bisque is a completely new turn. You should remember this when you take a bisque because it means that you are allowed to roquet all three balls again even though you haven't yet run a hoop.

Example 3
One of your balls, yellow, is in the middle of the lawn, while red is in corner three. With red, which is for hoop one, you shoot at blue (which is close to black near corner two) and hit. With a stop shot you send blue to hoop two. You then roquet black and send it to hoop one. With your continuation shot you put red close to blue (or yellow, it doesn't matter, but blue is closer). Your turn ends, but you have a bisque. Take the bisque and you start a new turn with the balls all laid out in a perfect four-ball break!

Bisque turns may be taken in sequence, so one bisque turn can immediately follow another.

Example 4
Having set up the four-ball break in example 3, you stick in hoop one. If you have several bisques, you can take a second one to continue through hoop one, maintaining the break.

What is my handicap?

The aim of any handicapping system is to give everyone an equal chance of winning. Croquet clubs have an appointed handicapper who tries to achieve this, but friends and families need to have their own system. A suggested system is described next. Note that the scheme is only intended for singles play; it is not really possible to decide individual handicapping in a doubles match.

Start off the system by giving everyone a handicap of ten. After each game, reduce the winner's handicap by one and increase the loser's handicap by one.

Example 5
ROY plays BOB in the first game. They are both ten. ROY beats BOB. ROY's handicap is now nine, BOB's is eleven. The next time they play, BOB will have a bisque advantage over ROY. If BOB wins this time they will both go back to ten. If ROY wins again, the handicaps will be eight and twelve respectively.

After a while, the wins and losses will probably even out as each player reaches his or her correct handicap. At this point it is not a good idea to change both handicaps after every game, but only reduce someone who wins two games in succession or increase someone who loses two games in succession.

If someone is really good and keeps winning even when their handicap reaches 0, just keep going into minus figures. Note that the difference between, say, minus two and twelve is fourteen, not ten.

How many bisques do I get?

There are two ways of calculating the number of bisques.

1   Standard handicap play

In this scheme, the higher handicap player receives bisques equal to the handicap difference of the players. So if ROY is seven and BOB is ten, BOB has three extra bisque turns.

This means that in the very first game, where everyone is ten, play will be level and there are no extra bisque turns for the two players.

Example 5
ROY plays BOB in the first game. They are both ten so play level. ROY beats BOB. ROY's handicap is now nine, BOB's is eleven. The next time they play, BOB will have two extra bisque turns' advantage over ROY. If BOB wins this time they will both go back to ten. If ROY wins again, the handicaps will be eight and twelve respectively and BOB will have four extra bisque turns next time they play.

2   Full bisque handicap play

In this scheme, each player receives bisques equal to his or her handicap.

So if ROY was seven and BOB was ten, ROY would have seven extra bisque turns and BOB would have ten extra bisque turns.

This will mean that in the very first game, each player has ten extra bisque turns.

Example 6
ROY plays BOB in the first game. They are both ten so each has ten extra bisque turns. ROY beats BOB. ROY's handicap is now nine, BOB's is eleven. The next time they play, BOB will have eleven extra bisque turns, while ROY will have nine. If BOB wins this time they will both go back to ten. If ROY wins again, they will have eight and twelve extra bisque turns respectively.

Which is the best scheme?

There are advantages and disadvantages to both schemes.

The standard scheme allows the better player to play without bisques and win on his or her own merits. Apart from the extra turns that the weaker player gets, the game is very close to a non-handicap match. However, it can take a long time to play a game to a conclusion without time limits, as already mentioned. Also, the better player is forced to play more defensively because of the extra turns that the opponent possesses.

The full bisque version allows both players to build breaks and get out of trouble. Constructive play is encouraged due to both sides having extra turns. The game should therefore be quicker. However, it is a more artificial situation as players know they can take risks that they would not take without bisques.

Faults

If a turn stops due to a fault being committed, for example sending a ball off court in a croquet stroke, a bisque can be used to start a new turn.

If bisque(s) are taken in a series of consecutive turns which then turn out to be invalid (for example, hoops scored in the wrong order), any bisques used after the error was committed are restored, but not any used before.

Doubles play

Although doubles play cannot be used to judge singles handicaps, players' handicaps can be used to play handicap doubles games.

For standard handicap doubles play the players of each pair add together their handicaps. The higher handicap side receives half the difference between the totals, rounded up to the nearest whole. Either player of a side may use the bisques.

Example 7
BOB (six) and ROY (five) play BOG (ten) and POW (four) (who normally play with the secondary colours!) in a handicap game.

BOB-ROY's total is eleven, BOG-POW's fourteen. BOG-POW therefore receive half of fourteen minus eleven, which is one and a half. This is rounded up to two.

For full bisque play, each player receives half their normal bisques, rounded up to the nearest whole. Players may only use their own bisques.

Example 8
Same match as example 7. BOB has three bisques, ROY has three bisques, BOG has five bisques and POW has two bisques.

If a player commits a fault and the turn ends, a bisque may be taken to start a new turn but only by the player who committed the fault.

Handicap tactics

This is a topic large enough for a book (see the Bibliography on page 131). Here are a few pointers to start you on the fascinating trail of tactical handicap croquet.

If you have a lot of bisques (six or more), use a couple to set up a four-ball break, plus others as necessary to maintain the break. Do not try this until you have enough skill to fulfil the elements of a four-ball break; see Chapter 5.

If you have a few bisques (three to five), look for situations where you can set up a three or four-ball break with just one bisque, then use others as necessary to maintain the break.

If you have one or two bisques, look for situations where you can set up a three or four-ball break with just one bisque.

Occasionally you should use a bisque defensively to get out of trouble, for example when you have failed to run a hoop and left your opponent a very easy break. However, remember that in a full bisque game, your opponent has bisques as well, so a purely defensive bisque may not be enough.

Do not use bisques for impossible or highly speculative situations, for the result will be a wasted bisque.

When faced with a difficult situation, consider if you can improve it with a bisque. If you can, remember that you can roquet all of the balls again, so you may be able to improve the situation even more than at first seemed possible.

If you have a situation which is possible but difficult by taking a bisque, consider if two bisques taken consecutively will make things easy.

When your opponent has bisques and you do not, do not leave situations that make it easy for him or her. Examples are:

- Leaving your balls near your opponent's hoop.

- Leaving a ball or balls near your opponent's next hoop.

- Leaving your balls in the middle of the lawn.

When your opponent has bisques and you do not, try to leave situations that encourage him or her to use bisques without good effect – in other words, waste them. Examples are:

- Leaving your balls with a rush for your hoop, but a long way from your opponent's hoop.

- Leaving a ball or balls near your hoops, but not your opponent's.

- Leaving your opponent's balls in the middle of the lawn, some way apart.

Doubles handicap tactics

Doubles play is not very different from singles play, but there are a few things to observe:

Discuss with your partner which is the best thing to do, but don't spend ages about it, or the game will get boring.

Having decided what to do, accept what happens, right or wrong. Do not argue about what might have been.

Watch your partner, and forestall any errors, but do not leap on court every two minutes to challenge or discuss play.

You can assist your partner in every way except with the actual shot. So you can line up balls and demonstrate swings, etc.

You should now have a working knowledge of basic croquet. Quite often, unusual points of law will occur in your games. To help with this, the next chapter gives a comprehensive reference guide to the rules of association croquet.

8

THE LAWS OF
—— ASSOCIATION ——
CROQUET

The official laws of croquet are published by the Croquet Association and may be obtained from them; see Appendix 1. They are complex, particularly when dealing with a version called 'advanced croquet'. This chapter is based on the 1989 edition, and rules have been simplified or amended where required. For those readers who possess the laws book and would like to cross-refer to it, this chapter uses the same numbers for the laws. This means that there will be missing numbers where laws that are not relevant to this book are omitted.

———— Guide to the laws ————

The laws are set out in a logical order. They start with a general description of the game, followed by detailed descriptions of specific actions such as roquets, hoop points and so on. Laws relating to things that can go wrong then follow. The final set of laws relates to variations of the standard game.

The list which follows will assist you in finding specific topics.

Topic and related laws

—————————— **Part 1** ——————————

The standard court and equipment

1 The standard court

This is a rectangle measuring 35 by 28 yards (32 by 25.6 metres). Where marking (a white line or string) is used, the inner edge is the exact boundary. Fig. 34 shows the measurements for a standard court.

2 Equipment

The peg should be 1½ inches (38mm) wide and 18 inches (450mm) high. It should have a detachable extension to hold clips.

Hoops should be 12 inches (300mm) high and between 3¾ inches (95mm) and 4 inches (100mm) wide.

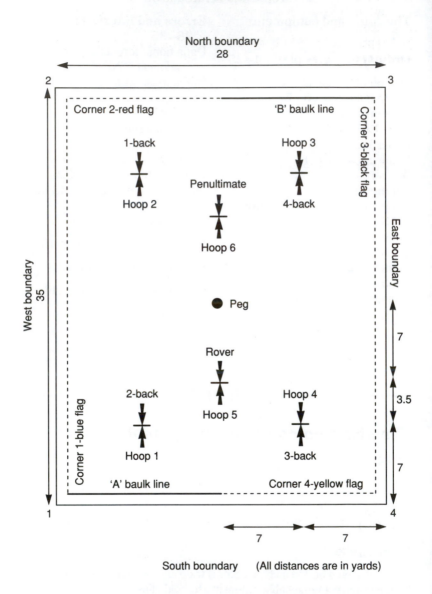

North boundary
28

Corner 2-red flag

'B' baulk line

Corner 3-black flag

1-back

Hoop 2

Penultimate

Hoop 3

4-back

Hoop 6

West boundary
35

East boundary

● Peg

Rover

2-back

Hoop 5

Hoop 4

Hoop 1

3-back

Corner 1-blue flag

'A' baulk line

Corner 4-yellow flag

7

3.5

7

7

7

South boundary   (All distances are in yards)

Fig. 34: The standard court

Balls should be 3⅝ inches (92mm) in diameter and weigh one pound (454kg). If they are coloured blue, black, red and yellow, blue/black plays red/yellow. If they are coloured green, brown, pink and white, green/brown plays pink/white. For other colours, the darker two balls play the lighter two.

Clips should be the same colour as the balls used. If no clips are available, painted clothes pegs will often suffice.

3 Court accessories

Flags and corner pegs are not essential to the game, but where provided may be placed as shown in fig. 35.

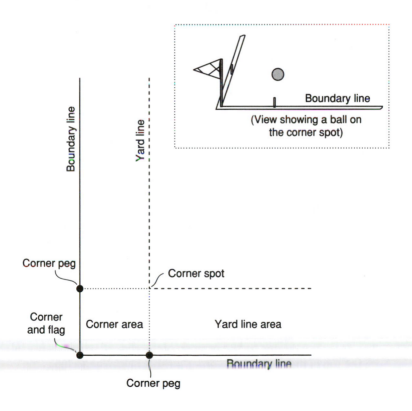

Fig. 35: The corner area

—————————— Part 2 ——————————

Ordinary singles play

4   An outline of the game

(a) This law describes the game generally and is modified by the detailed laws which follow.

(b) The object of the game is for a player – with both balls – to run all hoops in the correct sequence and then strike the peg.

A ball which has run all hoops but not yet struck the peg is called a rover ball. A rover ball which strikes the peg is then known as a pegged out ball. A pegged out ball is removed from the game. A rover ball can also cause any other rover ball to be pegged out (see law 15).

(c) The game is played by striking a ball with a mallet (see laws 31 and 32). The player whose turn it is, is known as the striker. The ball he or she strikes is the striker's ball. His or her other ball is the partner ball. The remaining two balls are the opponent's balls.

(d) Players play alternate turns. At the start of a turn a player chooses which ball to play (see law 8), and must strike only that ball in that turn (see law 28).

If the striker's ball runs a hoop, the striker is entitled to an extra stroke called a continuation stroke (see laws 4g and 21).

If the striker's ball makes a roquet (see law 16), the striker is entitled to two extra strokes. The first is known as a croquet stroke (see laws 4f and 20). It is played after placing the striker's ball in contact with the roqueted ball (see law 19). The second extra stroke is a continuation stroke, as described in 4g.

At the start of a turn the striker's ball may roquet each of the other three balls once only. If, however, a hoop is scored, the three balls may be roqueted once again.

(e) The score is indicated by the position of the clips. Each clip is placed on the top of the hoop next in order for that ball. When a full game is played (see Chapter 7), the clips are placed on the side of the hoop to indicate the second six hoops.

(f) In a croquet stroke the other ball must move or shake when the striker's ball is struck. Also, neither ball may go off court (see law 20).

(g) A continuation stroke is played in the same way as is the first stroke of a turn: i.e. a hoop may be run, a roquet made, etc. Continuation strokes are not cumulative, so:

- If a hoop and a roquet are made in the same stroke, croquet is taken and the hoop continuation shot is lost.

- If a roquet is made in a croquet stroke, croquet is taken and the continuation shot is lost.

- If two hoops are run in one stroke, only one continuation shot is allowed.

- If a hoop is made in a croquet stroke, only one continuation shot is allowed.

5   The toss

The winner of the toss may choose either to play first or second, or which colour balls to use. The loser has whichever choice is left.

6   The start of a game

At the start of the game, all four balls are played from any point on the 'A' or 'B' baulk lines. In the first turn the first player will play one of the chosen two balls. In the second turn the second player will do likewise. In the third and fourth turns the third and fourth balls *must* be brought into play. After this, law 4d applies.

7   Ball in play

Law 6 brings balls into play. Balls remain in play until pegged out and are eligible to score points, except under law 9.

8   Election of striker's ball

Law 4d allows the striker to choose a ball to play. This choice is indicated by either moving, lifting or striking a ball.

9   Ball in hand

Any ball is 'in hand' (and is not in play) when it is off court, or when it is in the yard line area at the end of a turn.

Additionally, the striker's ball is in hand when it has made a roquet. *Note:* this means that having made a roquet, the striker's ball cannot then bounce off and score a hoop or the peg, although it can score a point for another ball by peeling it (see laws 14f and 18).

10   Ball off court

A ball is off court when any part of it crosses over the inside edge of the boundary (see law 12).

11   Balls in the yard line area

All balls which do not go off court but end up in the yard line area are immediately placed on the yard line or corner spot as appropriate (see law 12). *Exception:* after a croquet stroke or having run a hoop, the striker's ball is not replaced but played from where it lies.

12   Replacement of balls off court or in the yard line area

Balls are replaced on the yard line at the nearest point to where the ball went off court (or lies if it stopped in the yard line area). If the ball went off, or lies, in the corner area (see fig. 35), it is replaced on the corner spot.

In all cases, if there is a ball already occupying the replacement spot, the striker's ball is replaced in contact with it, on the yard line. The striker chooses which side. Both balls must be on the yard line.

13   Wiring lift

At the start of a turn, if a striker's ball has no clear shot at any other ball, the striker may lift that ball and play it from the 'A' or 'B' baulk. A clear shot means being able to hit any part of the target ball with any part of the striker's ball.

These three conditions must also be met:

- The opponent must have put the striker's ball there.

- The obstruction(s) can only be hoops or the peg, not other balls.

- The striker's ball must not already be touching another ball (see law 16c).

A lift is also given, even when there is a clear shot, provided that the three conditions above are met and either the striker's backswing is impeded by a hoop or peg, or the striker's ball is in the jaws of a hoop.

14 Hoop point

(a) A ball scores a hoop point by passing through the correct hoop in the correct direction.

(b) The part of the hoop which faces the striker as he or she is about to run the hoop is called the playing side.

(c) A ball starts to run a hoop when its leading edge is level with the front of the hoop on the non-playing side. A ball completes the running of a hoop when its trailing edge no longer protrudes on the playing side.

(d) A ball may run a hoop in more than one turn; i.e. having started to run in one turn, it can complete in another.

(e) A hoop may be scored in a croquet stroke provided it has not begun to run the hoop when placed for that croquet stroke. See also law 4g.

(f) A ball other than the striker's ball can be made to score its hoop. This can occur in a croquet stroke (peeling) or in a roquet (rush peeling).

15 Peg point

Only a rover ball may score a peg point. When the point is scored, the ball is removed from the game. A rover ball may croquet or rush another rover ball onto the peg to peg it out. *Note:* In a rush peg out the turn ends because the rushed ball, although roqueted, is removed from the game.

16 Roquet

Definition
A roquet is made when the striker's ball hits one of the other three balls. A croquet stroke (see law 20) is then taken. From the start of a turn each of the three balls may, if desired, be roqueted in turn. If, meanwhile, a hoop is run, all balls roqueted so far may be roqueted again. No ball can be roqueted twice in the same turn unless a hoop is run.

Additional points
(a) The striker's ball can either make a roquet with a direct hit, or after it has hit a hoop or peg or another ball on which a roquet has already been made.

(b) If two balls are hit in the same shot, it is the first ball hit which is roqueted.

(c) If, at the start of a turn, the striker elects to play a ball that is in contact with another ball, a roquet is deemed to have been made and the striker takes croquet from that ball immediately.

(d) If there is another ball in the jaws of the striker's hoop, which may be, and is, roqueted, croquet is taken from that ball wherever it is rushed to. No hoop point is scored for the striker's ball even if it then continues through the hoop.

(e) If there is another ball in the jaws of the striker's hoop which has already been roqueted, a hoop point is scored if the striker's ball hits that ball and then continues through the hoop. No roquet is made except under (c) above.

17 Hoop and roquet in the same stroke

If there is a ball the other side of the hoop (clear of the jaws), which is hit as, or after, the striker's ball runs its hoop, hoop and roquet are scored together. Croquet is taken and the hoop continuation shot is lost. To achieve both hoop and roquet, when the striker's ball comes to rest, it must have passed through the hoop. If it has not, the hoop is not run and either croquet is taken if the other ball has not been roqueted before, or the turn ends if it has.

18 Consequences of a roquet

If a roquet is made, the striker's ball (in that stroke) cannot score a hoop or peg point for itself (except under law 17), but can cause other balls to score by knocking them through their hoop (rush peeling) or against the peg if they are rover balls (rush peg out).

19 Placing balls for the croquet stroke

(a) The striker's ball is placed in contact with the roqueted ball but not touching any other ball. It may touch a hoop or the peg but see law 32.

(b) If there are three balls (the striker's ball, the roqueted ball and one other) together on the yard line or in the corner, paragraph (a) applies plus: the third ball is then placed anywhere in contact with the roqueted ball but not in contact with the striker's ball.

(c) If there are four balls (the striker's ball, the roqueted ball and two others) together on the yard line or in the corner, paragraphs (a) and (b) apply plus: the fourth ball is then placed anywhere in contact with any ball except the striker's.

20 Croquet stroke

(a) In a croquet stroke the roqueted ball becomes known as the croqueted ball.

(b) The striker plays a stroke with the balls placed according to law 19 in such a way as to move or shake both balls.

(c) The striker's turn ends if, in the croquet stroke, either ball is sent off court. *Exception:* for the striker's ball only, the turn does not end if a roquet is made, or a hoop or peg point is scored before going off court.

21 Continuation stroke

The striker is entitled to a continuation stroke after a hoop point is scored. A continuation stroke is also taken after a croquet stroke except when the turn ends, see law 20c, or a roquet is made on another ball.

22 Ball moving between strokes

If a ball moves between a stroke or a turn, having previously come to rest, it is replaced and the game continues. No point is scored or lost by this movement.

23 Imperfections on the surface of the court

Loose items, for example twigs or leaves, may be removed before a stroke.

Balls may be lifted out of bad holes, ruts, etc. Any such movement should not give an advantage to the striker. This may mean the movement of other balls by an equal amount to give a similar shot. In the case of a hoop attempt, it may mean moving the ball further away from the hoop.

24 Interference with a stroke

If a fixed object such as a wall or tree impedes a shot, balls may be moved subject to the same conditions as rule 23.

25 Local laws

If a lawn is to be used for an official Croquet Association event, any special conditions must be approved by the Association. For clubs or individuals, special conditions may be applied as seen fit.

Errors and interference in play

26 Definitions

Forestalling
An opponent or partner forestalls when the striker is stopped from playing due to an error or fault which has been, or is about to be, committed.

Limit of claims
This is the time after which forestalling has no effect, i.e. there is no specific remedy for the error.

Condoning
Any error or fault spotted after the limit of claims is condoned, i.e. it is allowed to stand without correction. Where there is the phrase 'Condoned if not noticed by . . .', it is followed by the limit of claims for that error or fault.

27 Playing when not entitled to do so

Examples are: playing when it is not your turn; taking croquet twice from the same ball in the same turn without running a hoop; and continuing to play having run the wrong hoop. Any such play is invalid. Balls and clips are returned to their original positions. However, such invalid play is condoned if not noticed before the first stroke of the next player's turn.

28 Playing a wrong ball

If the striker strikes either of the opponent balls, or changes to the partner ball in the middle of a turn, balls and clips are replaced in their original positions before the wrong ball was struck and the striker's turn ends. Playing a wrong ball is condoned if not noticed before the first stroke of the next player's turn.

29 Playing when a ball is misplaced – general rule

In the following situations, a ball is misplaced. If noticed, the ball(s) are replaced correctly and play continues without penalty. Misplacement is condoned if not noticed before the stroke is played.

(a) A ball incorrectly placed after the end of the previous turn.

(b) A ball wrongly brought back onto the yard line (see law 11).

(c) A ball wrongly left in the yard line area or off court.

(d)   Not playing a ball from a baulk line when it should have been.

(e)   Playing a croquet stroke when the balls are not touching, or the striker's ball is touching a ball other than the croqueted ball.

(f)   Anything else not covered by law 30.

30   Playing when a ball is misplaced – exceptions

The exceptions are:

(a) Taking croquet from a wrong ball.

(b) Taking croquet from a ball which has not yet been roqueted.

(c) Not taking croquet when roquet has been made.

(d) Wrongly removing or failing to remove a ball from the game.

In all cases, the balls are replaced to their positions before the error and the striker continues without penalty, playing the correct shot. The difference between these exceptions and the general rule is that they are condoned if not noticed before the *next stroke but one* of the striker's turn.

31   Definition of a stroke and the striking period

A stroke is any movement of the mallet which is intended to strike the ball (even if it does not actually do so). Practice swings are not strokes. A stroke ends when all balls stop moving.

The striking period starts at the beginning of a stroke and ends when the striker quits his stance (this may be before or after the end of the stroke).

Note: a player may leave a ball where it is and deem a stroke to have been played.

32   Faults

The following are faults which may be made *during the striking period*. In each case, balls and clips are replaced to their original positions before the fault was committed and the striker's turn ends. They are condoned if not noticed before the next stroke but one of the striker's turn.

(a)   Touching the mallet head with the hand.

(b)   Kicking or hitting the mallet onto the ball.

(c)   Resting the mallet shaft, or a hand or arm, on the ground or the striker's legs or feet.

(d) Not striking the ball with the end-face of the mallet.

(e) Steering or pushing a ball, i.e. maintaining contact with it.

(f) Striking a ball more than once, except when making a roquet or pegging out.

(g) Touching any ball other than the striker's with the mallet.

(h) Touching any ball with anything other than the mallet.

(i) Crushing the striker's ball against a hoop or the peg. To be a crush, hoop, ball and mallet must be in contact at the same time (except when striking away from an obstruction).

(j) In a croquet stroke, not moving or shaking the croqueted ball. If this fault is committed and the striker's ball also goes off court (law 20c), the opponent may choose which error and consequent remedy applies.

The following is also a fault, with the same conditions as the above, but only when a shot is hampered.

(k) Striking the ball with the bevelled edge of the mallet face.

A shot is hampered if a hoop, ball or peg interferes with a normal shot (single ball or croquet). (It should be noted that although faults (b) to (i) can occur anywhere, they are more likely to do so in a hampered shot. Special care should therefore be taken and in the absence of an independent observer or referee, the opponent should be invited to watch the shot for faults.) *Note:* It is not a fault to strike the ball with the bevelled edge of the mallet in an unhampered shot, but this should never be done deliberately.

33 Interference with a ball between strokes

A ball that is so moved is replaced without penalty.

34 Interference with a ball during a stroke

(a) By the striker. It is a fault under law 32 if the interference occurs during the striking period (see law 31). Otherwise the ball is replaced without penalty.

(b) By anyone or anything else. The ball is replaced without penalty. If the ball was moving at the time, it is placed where it would have gone unless the shot was critical, for example an attempt to make a roquet, which may or may not have hit, in which case it is replayed.

35 Playing when misled

If the striker is misled because the opponent has placed the clips incorrectly, or gives false information, a replay is permitted. The replay starts from the point where the striker was first misled. The replay must not be a repeat of the original turn as the striker could not then claim to have been misled.

—————————— **Part 3** ——————————

Other forms of play: handicap play

38 Bisques

Definition
A bisque is an extra turn. It is taken directly after the end of the striker's current turn. A bisque turn must be taken using the same ball that was used in the previous turn. Bisque turns may be taken in sequence, i.e. one bisque turn can immediately follow another.

Number
The number of bisques to be given is as follows:

(a) For standard handicap play, the higher handicap player receives bisques equal to the handicap difference of the players.

(b) For full bisque handicap play, each player receives bisques equal to his or her handicap.

It is common to use small sticks to indicate the number of bisques left.

Faults
If a turn ends due to a fault being committed, a bisque can be used to start a new turn.

Restoration of bisques
If bisque(s) are taken in a series of consecutive turns which then turn out to be invalid and are not condoned (for example, hoops scored in the wrong order), any bisques used in error are restored.

Other forms of play: doubles play

40 General

Outline of the game
The game is played between two sides of two players. Each player has one ball and may strike only that ball.

Assistance to partner
One partner may assist the other in any way except in the actual playing of strokes or standing as a line-of-sight marker.

For doubles, the rules of singles apply, substituting 'partner's ball' for 'partner ball'. Also 'player' includes 'side' and 'striker' includes 'striker's partner'.

43 Handicap doubles play

Number of bisques to be given
(a) For standard handicap doubles play each side adds together their handicap. The higher handicap side receives half the difference between the totals, rounded up to the nearest whole. Either player of a side may use the bisques.

(b) For full bisque play, each player receives half their normal bisques, rounded up to the nearest whole. Players may only use their own bisques.

Faults
If a player commits a fault and the turn ends, a bisque may be taken to start a new turn but only by the player that committed the fault (except in alternate stroke doubles).

Alternate stroke doubles play
This is played in the same way as standard doubles except that each player of a partnership plays each stroke alternately. This alternation always occurs, even after faults and bisques. The second sentence of law 40 does not apply.

44 Customs of the game

Croquet relies heavily on the honesty of players. Faults and errors must be announced, even when not spotted by the opponent. Situations where faults might occur should be noted and if necessary watched by an independent observer (where available) or opponent.

The opponent should watch the game but does not have to. However, by not watching, a fault may pass the limit of claims, see law 26.

Normally, potential faults should be forestalled before they occur. Specifically however, playing a wrong ball and running a wrong hoop should only be forestalled after the fault has occurred (note that running a wrong hoop is not a fault but taking a continuation stroke afterward is).

Players should not spend too long between each shot; expedition is called for . . .

No artificial aids to play are allowed.

51   Emergency law

Situations not appearing to be covered by these laws should be dealt with as fairly as can be arranged.

9

—— FUN GAMES ——

Although croquet is a game to be enjoyed, it does require serious concentration to play it properly. The games described in this chapter are much simpler. They can be played for the odd half hour before lunch, or to relax after a concentrated game of croquet.

In all the games described, play is sequential as in golf croquet (see Chapter 3). Also, all balls which go off court or in the yard line area are replaced on the yard line.

—————— Four-ball ——————

A game for two or four players.

This is a similar game to golf croquet. The rules are the same as golf croquet with the following additions:

1   You gain an extra shot by either running a hoop, or hitting another ball with yours (making a roquet).

Note: The extra shot you gain by making a roquet is played from where your ball lies. You do not take croquet. Like association croquet, you can only roquet each of the other balls once before running a hoop.

2   If you hit two balls in the same shot, it is the first one hit that is roqueted. You are then allowed to hit the other one if you want to.

3   If you stick in the jaws of a hoop, you are allowed (if still there) to continue through next turn.

Robber

A game for any number of players.

1 Start anywhere on the yard line.

2 You can run any hoop in any direction. Each time that you do so, you score one point. You do not get an extra shot for running a hoop.

3 If you roquet another player's ball, you 'rob' him or her of their points. You also gain one extra shot (as in four-ball, you do not take croquet).

4 Each time you reach ten points, these are 'banked' and cannot be stolen.

For example: ROY has six points and roquets BOB who has seven points. ROY now has thirteen points and BOB has none. BOB now roquets ROY. ROY has banked ten points, so only loses three. ROY now has ten points and BOB has three.

5 The first player to reach 31 is the winner (this figure can be altered to suit the time available).

Tag

A game for three to six players.

The object of the game is to catch up with your opponents and 'tag' them, removing them from the game. The last player left is the winner.

1 Draw lots for the order of play. Alternatively, play in order of hitting ability, strongest last.

2 Players start one yard in front of their starting hoop.

3 Starting hoops are as follows:

For three players –

player one – hoop one; player two – hoop two; player three – hoop five.

For four players –

player one – hoop one; player two – hoop four; player three – hoop one-back; player four – hoop four-back.

For five players –

player one – hoop one; player two – hoop three; player three – hoop six; player four – hoop two-back; player five – hoop four-back.

For six players –

player one – hoop one; player two – hoop three; player three – hoop five; player four – hoop one-back; player five – hoop three-back; player six – penultimate hoop.

4   The route is circular and continuous. For three players the route is hoop one to six and back to hoop one again (a six-hoop loop). For four to six players the route is hoop one to rover and back to hoop one again (a twelve-hoop loop).

5   You must run hoops in a single turn. A ball stuck in a hoop can be played in either direction next turn but does not score the hoop.

6   If you run a hoop you continue your turn by one extra shot. If you run two hoops in the same stroke, you have two extra shots.

7   You may 'tag', i.e. roquet, any ball which is for the same hoop as you. Also, that ball can tag yours. Any ball which is tagged is removed from the game. Tagging gives one extra shot.

For example, at the start of a game for six players, ROY (player one) runs hoop one. The ball stops two yards from hoop two. With the continuation stroke he runs hoop two. He is now for the same hoop as player two who is in front of hoop three. He can shoot at player two. If he hits, he has tagged that player, who is removed from the game. He will also earn a further continuation shot. If he misses, he will end up close to player two who may then tag him.

He therefore does not have to shoot, but may lurk somewhere, waiting for his chance.

8   It is quite possible for players to overtake one another. A player who overtakes cannot tag the one overtaken as they are now for different hoops. The order of play remains the same.

9   If you tag a ball which is not for the same hoop, you miss the next turn and any extra shots earned for this turn.

One-ball

A game for two players.

The rules are exactly the same as for association croquet except that each player has only one ball.

Despite this rather short description, one-ball is a good game, with some interesting tactics, especially when both players are going for the same hoop. Try it and discover them for yourself!

10

—— JOINING A CLUB ——

As your game improves you will want to try your skills out against other players. The best way to do this is to join a croquet club. Here you will find a friendly atmosphere and a chance to play on full-size lawns.

If you do not know the location of your nearest club, try your local library. If they do not know, the best way to find out is to contact your national croquet association. Their addresses are given in Appendix 1.

Many clubs will have a coaching programme for beginners and improvers. You will find that having read and understood this book, you will already be well on the way to being considered an improver.

From here on, you can go as far as your ability and inclination will take you. You can simply play friendly games at your club, enjoying the company and the relaxation, or, if you want a little more competition, most clubs have a selection of events throughout the season which cater for differing abilities.

The larger clubs also run weekend and even week-long tournaments. If you want to enter these you should, if you haven't already done so, join your croquet association (see below).

Your next step upwards is to improve your play to such a standard that you will play advanced rules croquet, mentioned very briefly in this book. You can then play in advanced play tournaments, championships and, who knows, represent your country in international events.

——— Croquet associations ———

Each country where croquet is played has an organisation which acts as national representative for that country. In most cases it is called 'The Croquet Association of . . .' (followed by the country). The purpose of such an association is to act as a central body to promote and regulate croquet for that country. It will organise competitions from individual to international level. It will have membership or representation on the World Croquet Council. Affiliation to or membership of your association is very much to be encouraged because you will not only receive the benefits of membership – magazines, tournament opportunities, etc – you will be contributing to the continuance of your chosen sport.

Some associations run special events for newcomers. Where known, they are listed in the following appendix. Your association will also be able to put you in touch with your nearest club.

—— APPENDIX 1 ——

Addresses of Croquet Associations

World

Secretary-General,
Mr Chris Hudson,
The Oaklands,
Englesea Brook,
Near Crewe,
Cheshire, CW2 5QW,
England.

Australia

Mrs C N Fox,
Hon Secretary,
Australian Croquet Association,
PO Box 296,
Rosney Park,
Tasmania 7018.

Nationally, events for beginners are under review. Each state also has its own association, with state-oriented tournaments.

Canada

Croquet Canada,
PO Box 892,
60 James Street,
St Catherines,
Ontario, L2R 6Z4.

England

The Secretary,
The Croquet Association,
The Hurlingham Club,
Ranelagh Gardens,
London, SW6 3PR.

England is also divided into nine regions, each with its own local federation council.

There are three national events for newcomers to croquet.

The Croquet Classic
This event is open to any player in England and Wales who has never had a handicap less than 19. It is a national event aimed specifically at garden croquet players. Preliminary rounds can sometimes be held on your own lawn. To find out details, contact the English Croquet Association.

The Golden Mallet Competition
This is a National Golf Croquet tournament open to any player who has never had a handicap less than 19. Preliminary rounds will be held locally. To find out details, contact the English Croquet Association.

National Schools Championship
This tournament is designed to encourage croquet within schools. Teams of three compete in leagues, the winners of which go forward to regional, then national, finals.

Finland

Ylöjärven Krokettiklubi,
Soppeenmäen Keskuskenttä,
Hämeenpuisto 14 A 8,
33210 Tampere.

France

Federation Française de Croquet,
4 Quai Victor Hugo,
85200 Fontenay-Le-Compte.

Guernsey

King George V playing fields.

Ireland

The Secretary,
The Croquet Association of Ireland,
c/o Carrickmines Croquet & Lawn Tennis Club,
Carrickmines,
Dublin 18.

The CAI holds a beginners tournament during the Championship of Ireland in July. Games take place under the supervision of an experienced player.

Isle of Man

Ann Cottier,
Yn Clyst,
36 Victoria Road,
Castletown, IOM.

The Manx Croquet Association holds an open singles and doubles event, the Manx Classic, in May each year.

Italy

Associazione Italiana Croquet,
Segretaria Generale,
CP 367,
21052 Busto Arsizio (VA).

A tournament for beginners is being considered.

Japan

The Croquet Association of Japan,
4-6-16,
Matsushiro,
Tsukuba,
Ibaraki, 305.

A croquet-like game called 'Gate-Ball' is also played in Japan.

Jersey

Jersey Croquet Club,
Les Quennevais Playing Fields,
St Brelade.

Kenya

H A Curtis,
PO Box 10,
Limuru.

New Zealand

The National Secretary,
The New Zealand Croquet Council, Inc,
PO Box II-259,
Wellington.

Organised coaching available to beginners.

Scotland

Hon Secretary,
13 Park Place,
Dunfermline,
Fife, KY12 7QL.

The SCA holds occasional courses for beginners.

South Africa

The Secretary,
South African Croquet Association,
PO Box 259
Constantia 7848.

Switzerland

Association Suisse de Croquet,
Peter J Payne,
En Molard-Rochau,
1261 Genolier.

Sweden

Svenska Croquetförbundet,
c/o Fred Sandström,   or Ian Insulander,
Elsaborgsgata 50,   Hasselstigen 38,
S-12665 Hägersten.   S-15230 Südertälje.

Courses for beginners can often be arranged on request to the association.

United States

There are a number of different versions of croquet played in the USA. Association croquet is played extensively in the west, under the auspices of the American Croquet Association.

In the east, the United States Croquet Association has its own rules. It is a sequence game with the 'yard line' being only nine inches. Although the basic strokes are the same as association croquet, this book is unsuitable for USCA rules croquet. Association rules games are, however, beginning to be played at some locations.

Anne Frost,
US Croquet Association,
500 Avenue of Champions,
Palm Beach Gardens,
Florida 33418.

United States garden croquet also tends to be played according to sequence rules, often with the old nine hoop, two peg setting.

Yet another croquet-like game is played throughout the States. This is called 'Roque'. It is played on a sandy court, ten yards by twenty, with a concrete surround, and with short-handled mallets. The headquarters are in Dallas, Texas.

In America a hoop is called a wicket and a peg is called a stake.

Wales

60 Coleridge Avenue,
Penarth,
South Glamorgan, CF6 1SQ.

The author also believes that croquet is, or has been, played in the Bahamas, Bermuda, Brazil, China, Costa Rica, Egypt, Indonesia, Jamaica, Mexico, the Netherlands, Portugal, Russia, Singapore, Spain and Tenerife.

Croquet may also be found at hotels, sports clubs and universities throughout the world – but you will probably have to ask for it!

APPENDIX 2

Addresses of Croquet Equipment Manufacturers

The Australian Croquet
Company,
1349 South Road,
Bedford Park, SA 5042
Australia

Natural Alternatives,
PO Box 2477,
Gravenhurst,
Ontario, POC 1G0
Canada

Sun Lucky Ltd,
Oimazato 3-13-6,
Higashinari-ku,
Osaka, 537
Japan

Jackson Mallets,
18 Caspar Rd,
Papatoetoe,
Auckland,
New Zealand

True-Line Croquet Equipment,
58 Wellington St,
Hamilton,
New Zealand

Barlow Balls,
Tom Barlow,
PO Box 1792,
Somerset West 7130
South Africa

John Jaques & Son Ltd,
361 Whitehorse Rd,
Thornton Heath,
Surrey, CR7 8XP
UK

Stortime Products,
Unit 14,
Southmill Trading Centre,
Southmill Road,
Bishops Stortford,
Herts, CM23 3DY
UK

Townsend Croquet Ltd,
Claire Rd,
Kirby Cross,
Frinton-on-Sea,
Essex, CO13 0LX
UK

Country Crafts,
Manor Cottage,
Widecombe in the Moor,
Devon, TQ13 7TB
UK

Woodlands Croquet Products,
Woodlands,
Skipton Rd,
Barnoldswick,
Colne, Lancs, BB8 6HH
UK

Manor House Croquet,
The Manor House,
1 Barn Croft,
Penwortham,
Preston, PR1 0SX
UK

Birkdale Croquet Equipment,
6 Walmer Road,
Birkdale,
Southport, PR8 4SX
UK

Croquet Department,
Forster Mfg Co Inc,
PO Box 657,
Wilton, ME 04294-0657
USA

Stanley Patmor,
4735 N 32PL,
Phoenix, AZ 85018
USA

—— BIBLIOGRAPHY ——

The following books are recommended by the author as good follow-on material to this book. Most are available from the English Croquet Association. The Australian, New Zealand, South African and United States associations also have their own books on sale.

The History of Croquet, by D M C Pritchard

An excellent book for those who would like to know more about the history of the game.

Plus One on Time, by D L Gaunt

A detailed look at handicap play and tactics, aimed at players in the medium to high handicap ranges.

Croquet, by J Solomon

Covers all aspects of the game up to advanced level.

Croquet, The Skills of the Game, by W Lamb

Gives a good insight into break-building techniques.

The CA Coaching Handbook

Although aimed at Croquet Association coaches, this book contains a lot of useful tips and exercises.

Laws of Croquet

The official rule book for association croquet.

Coaching Video by Joe Hogan (New Zealand)

Basic shots and techniques are demonstrated.

Croquet, Its History, Strategy, Rules and Records by J Charlton & W Thompson

This is a good beginner's guide to USCA rules croquet. It also contains sections on American garden croquet and the game of roque.

– GLOSSARY OF TERMS –

'A' baulk	See **baulk**.
Advanced rules	A version of croquet played at croquet tournaments which has extra rules to make the game more difficult for top level players.
Aiming point	The point at which to aim in a croquet stroke when it is required that the two balls are sent in different, and predicted, directions. Also the point at which to aim in an angled hoop shot.
'B' baulk	See **baulk**.
Baulk	A line, one yard in from the **boundary line**, along the **yard line**, stretching from the **corner spot** at corner one to half-way along the southern yard line (**'A' baulk**) and from the corner spot at corner three to half-way along the northern yard line (**'B' baulk**). Used when starting a game and for **lift** shots.
Bisque	An extra turn in a handicap game. Also the stick used to indicate the presence of such a turn or turns.
Boundary line	A line, of chalk, string, etc, forming the limits of the court. The inside edge of the boundary line forms the actual boundary.
Break	A turn containing more than one stroke. Sometimes referred to as an X-hoop break where X is the number of hoops scored in that turn. See also **two**, **three** and **four-ball breaks**.

Continuation stroke	An additional stroke which follows either a **croquet stroke** or **running a hoop**.
Corner	The joining points of the four **boundary lines**.
Corner area	Four one square-yard areas of the court. Their two outer edges are formed by the **boundary line**, one yard along from each **corner**. The two inner edges extend into the court and meet at the **corner spots**.
Corner spot	The innermost point of a **corner area**. A ball which goes off court one yard or less from a corner is replaced on the corner spot.
Croquet stroke	Striking your ball when it has been placed in contact with a **roqueted** ball.
Croqueted ball	The other ball (not your ball) in a croquet stroke. *Note:* before taking croquet, this ball was called the **roqueted ball**.
Crush	Forcing your ball against a hoop or the peg with your mallet. A crush is a **fault**.
Doubles	A game of croquet between four players, each playing one ball and playing as two pairs.
Double target	Two balls close to each other presenting a wide target to the striker. Three balls can form a triple target.
Drive shot	A croquet stroke played without **roll** or **stop** attributes.
Either ball rule	The rule which allows a player to choose which of the two balls is most advantageous to play. See also **sequence game**.
Error	Any action other than with the mallet which is contrary to the rules of croquet. Errors often incur a penalty. See also **fault**.
Fault	Any action with the mallet which is contrary to the rules of croquet. Most faults incur a penalty. The term foul is not used in croquet. See also **error**.

Four-ball break   A **break** using the striker's ball plus three others.

Free shot   A shot at a ball which, if missed, results in your ball going to a safe place on the court. See also **safe shot**.

Full game   A game in which the six hoops are run in both directions by both balls. A 26-point game.

Guarded leave   Finishing your turn by leaving your balls in such a way that if your opponent shoots at them and misses, you can make a **break** from the resulting situation.

Half angle   The way to calculate the **aiming point** for a **croquet stroke** which sends the two balls in different directions.

Hoop point   See **running a hoop**.

Innings   Control of the situation. A player who has such control is said to have the innings.

Jaws   The space between the uprights of a hoop.

Join up   Finishing a turn by leaving your balls close together. Careless joining up can leave a **double target**.

Lift shot   A rule by which a player may lift a ball and play it from **baulk**. A lift is given when an opponent **wires** the striker's ball.

Peel   Causing a ball other than the striker's ball to score a hoop point. If the peel occurs as a result of a **roquet** it is called a **rush peel**.

Peg out   The hitting of the peg by a ball which has scored all of its hoops. The ball is then known as a **pegged out ball**. It has completed the course and is removed from the game. The first player or side to peg out both balls is the winner.

Pegged out ball   See **peg out**.

Penultimate   The last but one hoop in a **full game**.

Pioneer	The ball sent to your next hoop but one in **three-** and **four-ball breaks**.
Pivot	The central ball in a **four-ball break**.
Push shot	A stroke in which the mallet maintains contact with the ball. This steers or pushes the ball rather than striking it. A push shot is a **fault**.
Roll shot	A **croquet stroke** in which both balls travel approximately the same distance.
Roquet	Hitting another ball with your own. A **croquet stroke** is then taken.
Roqueted ball	The ball that you have just hit. *Note:* when you play the **croquet stroke**, this ball becomes the **croqueted ball**.
Rover	A ball which has run all of its hoops. Also the name given to the final hoop of a game in a **full game**.
Running a hoop	Causing a ball to pass through its correct hoop in the correct direction. A ball which runs a hoop correctly scores a point, called a **hoop point**.
Rush	The movement of another ball which has been **roqueted**.
Rush peel	See **peel**.
Safe shot	A shot which gives little away if missed, even if your ball stops near an opponent ball.
Scatter	Striking your ball so that it hits another ball on which no **roquet** can be made.
Scoring a hoop	See **running a hoop**.
Sequence game	An old way of playing croquet in which balls were played in strict sequence. Still played in golf croquet. See also **either ball rule**.
Setting	Refers to the way that the hoops and peg are placed on a lawn. Also refers to the adjustment of a hoop to the correct width.

Singles A game of croquet between two players, each playing two balls.

Stalking The process of approaching your ball along the line of strike so that you take up the correct stance.

Stop shot A **croquet stroke** in which the striker's ball travels only a short distance compared with the other ball.

Take-off A **croquet stroke** in which the other ball stays virtually where it lies, while your ball is sent the required distance.

Taking croquet The act of placing two balls so as to play a **croquet stroke**.

Three-ball break A **break** using the striker's ball plus two others.

Tice A ball which is placed, usually at the beginning of a game, to tempt the opponent into shooting at it and missing.

Tie A game where the scores are equal after **time**. The game continues until one further point is scored.

Time Both the period allowed in a game limited by the clock and the call which indicates the reaching of that limit. See also **tie**.

Two-ball break A **break** using the striker's ball plus one other.

Wiring A ball is wired when a player cannot strike it so as to hit any other ball. If the wiring was caused by the opponent a player may claim a **lift shot**.

Yard line A line exactly one yard inside the **boundary line**. The line on which balls are replaced when they go out of court. The yard line is not normally marked.

Yard line area The area between the **yard line** and the **boundary line**.

OTHER TITLES AVAILABLE
IN TEACH YOURSELF

☐	0 340 56148 3	**Golf**	£4.99
		Bernard Gallacher and Mark Wilson	
☐	0 340 56779 1	**Walking and Rambling**	£5.99
		Heather MacDermid	
☐	0 340 55937 3	**Flower Arranging**	£6.99
		Judith Blacklock	
☐	0 340 32438 4	**Bridge**	£5.99
		Terence Reese	

*All these books are available at your local bookshop or newsagent, or can be ordered direct from
the publisher. Just tick the titles you want and fill in the form below.*

Prices and availability subject to change without notice.

HODDER AND STOUGHTON PAPERBACKS, P.O. Box 11, Falmouth, Cornwall.

Please send cheque or postal order for the value of the book, and add the following for
postage and packing:

UK including BFPO – £1.00 for one book, plus 50p for the second book, and 30p for each
additional book ordered up to a £3.00 maximum.

OVERSEAS, INCLUDING EIRE – £2.00 for the first book, plus £1.00 for the second
book, and 50p for each additional book ordered. OR Please debit this amount from my
Access/Visa Card (delete as appropriate).

Card Number

AMOUNT £ . . . .

EXPIRY DATE . . . .

SIGNED . . . .

NAME . . . .

ADDRESS . . . .

. . . .